Neuroimaging of Traumatic Brain Injury

Natalia Zakharova • Valery Kornienko
Alexander Potapov • Igor Pronin

Neuroimaging
of Traumatic Brain Injury

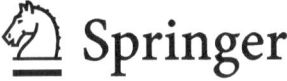

Natalia Zakharova, MD
Department of Neuroradiology
Burdenko Neurosurgery Intitute
Moscow
Russia

Valery Kornienko, MD
Department of Neuroradiology
Burdenko Neurosurgery Intitute
Moscow
Russia

Alexander Potapov, MD
Department of Neurotrauma
Burdenko Neurosurgery Insitute
Moscow
Russia

Igor Pronin, MD
Department of Neuroradiology
Burdenko Neurosurgery Institute
Moscow
Russia

ISBN 978-3-319-04354-8   ISBN 978-3-319-04355-5   (eBook)
DOI 10.1007/978-3-319-04355-5
Springer Cham Heidelberg New York Dordrecht London

Library of Congress Control Number: 2014933955

Printed on acid-free paper

Springer is part of Springer Science+Business Media (www.springer.com)

Preface

The main cause of severe traumatic brain injury worldwide is traffic accidents which are characterized by predominant acceleration-deceleration forces in various combinations with coup-contrecoup impact, thus making diffuse axonal injury (DAI) prevail in brain trauma alongside with focal and multifocal contusions and intracranial hemorrhages.

Until recently, no method has been developed for an accurate in vivo diagnosis of DAI and its severity due to poor differentiation of this type of injury by CT and conventional MRI. CT imaging has proved to be less sensitive to microstructural damage of the white matter, basal ganglia, internal capsule, thalamus, and brain stem if not accompanied by hemorrhages. Therefore, the implementation of more sensitive methods in DAI diagnostics in clinical practice is of primary importance.

The use of MRI in T2-FLAIR and T2* gradient echo impulse sequences and advanced modalities such as SWI and DWI has allowed a more accurate diagnosis and prognosis of outcome in TBI, depending on the severity and location of hemispheric and brain stem damage.

Application of the diffusion-tensor MRI (DT-MRI) has opened up new opportunities for a quantitative and qualitative evaluation of the white matter fiber tract injuries, obtaining their 3D images, and therefore, visualization of DAI severity in vivo.

However, dynamic evaluation of fiber tract destruction resulting in serious consciousness and mental disorders and sensory and motor dysfunction after TBI still remains unsolved. It is also not clear if DT-MRI is useful in identifying not only degeneration but regeneration of the brain during recovery process.

The assessment of regional cerebral blood flow (rCBF) disturbances is particularly important for understanding pathogenesis of TBI. Many scientists have been searching for clinically adequate methods of quantitative and qualitative evaluation of the rCBF. These methods have advantages and disadvantages and depend on such factors as availability, price-quality ratio, and patient safety.

CT perfusion is a relatively new method of minimally invasive quantitative mapping of the rCBF, which can be used in patients with different vascular or oncological pathology as well as traumatic brain injury.

However, the dominating patterns of regional CBF in hemispheric structures as well as in the brain stem have not been studied enough by the CT perfusion method in TBI patients.

Thus, it is important to investigate anatomical changes by various MRI impulse sequences and regional cerebral blood flow parameters by CT perfusion. Therefore, the main objective of this book is to facilitate the study of structural and hemodynamic brain changes in TBI using the results of clinical examinations and CT-MRI findings.

The book contains 6 chapters.

Chapter 1 reviews modern neuroimaging technologies and clarifies the main principles of recent diagnostic methods which allow better understanding of anatomical and pathophysiological changes in traumatic brain injury.

Clinical characteristics of the examined patients and neuroimaging methods are presented in Chap. 2.

In Chap. 3 we discuss the results of the study of correlation between severity, location, and level of hemispheric and brain stem damage based on clinical, CT, and MRI comparison analysis. A comprehensive MRI classification of localization of the brain stem and hemispheric structural damage has been proposed. This classification significantly correlates with Glasgow Coma Scale and Glasgow Outcome Scale, thus proving its prognostic value.

Chapter 4 is dedicated to dynamic structural changes of the white matter tracts examined by DT-MRI on the model of diffuse axonal injury. The new data on pathogenesis and dynamics of diffuse brain injury with quantitative and qualitative changes in the white matter fiber tracts have been obtained. It was demonstrated that DAI, being a trigger mechanism of fiber tract degeneration with their subsequent atrophy, may be regarded as a clinical model of multidimensional "split brain" with commissural (interhemispheric), association (intrahemispheric), and projection white matter tract disturbances.

In Chaps. 5 and 6 specific features of the regional hemispheric CBF and brain stem blood flow based on the dynamic CT perfusion studies in patients with focal and diffuse brain injuries are presented. Quantitative blood flow parameters in the brain stem using CT perfusion have been studied in comatose patients, with regard to dynamics of the traumatic brain disease and its outcome.

The developed indications for using various MRI sequences (T1, T2, T2-FLAIR, diffusion-weighted imaging (DWI), T2* gradient echo (SWAN), DT-MRI) and CT perfusion allow optimizing the diagnostic algorithm in severe TBI.

The comparison of clinical signs of trauma severity and outcome and qualitative and quantitative parameters of structural brain damage and cerebral blood flow changes helped us to identify significant criteria for clinical prognosis.

The classification developed for the brain injury localization and levels based on MRI data may become a useful tool for forming the databank on TBI, studying clinical comparative evaluation of efficacy of various approaches for the management of patients with severe TBI.

Moscow, Russia   Natalia Zakharova
                                                                      Valery Kornienko
                                                                   Alexander Potapov
                                                                           Igor Pronin

Acknowledgements

The authors would like to specially thank the colleagues from Burdenko Neurosurgery Institute who took part in this multidisciplinary study which made the basis for the presented monograph:

Alexandrova Eugenia, Arutyunov Nikita, Gavrilov Anton, Danilov Gleb, Dolgushin Mikhail, Eolchiyan Sergey, Zaitsev Oleg, Kravchuk Alexander, Likhterman Leonid, Melikyan Zara, Mikadze Yury, Oknina Lyubov, Okhlopkov Vladimir, Oshorov Andrey, Pestovskaya Natalia, Podoprigora Alexey, Polupan Alexander, Rodionov Pavel, Serkov Sergey, Sychev Alexander, Takush Sergey, Tenedieva Valeria, Turkin Alexander, Fadeeva Liudmila, Chelyapina Marina, Sharova Elena, and Shurkhay Vsevolod.

Our special thanks go to Professor Alexander Konovalov who helped this book on its way by constant support and advice.

Research supported by:

The Russian Foundation for Basic Research (RFBR), Grant number 13-04-12061

Abbreviations

ACA	Anterior cerebral artery
ADC	Apparent diffusion coefficient
AG	Angiography
CC	Corpus callosum
CPP	Cerebral perfusion pressure
CST	Corticospinal tract
CT	Computed tomography
DAI	Diffuse axonal injury
DTI	Diffusion tensor imaging
DWI	Diffusion weighted imaging
EDH	Epidural hematoma
FA	Fractional anisotropy
GCS	Glasgow Coma Scale
GOS	Glasgow Outcome Scale
ICH	Intracerebral hematoma
ICP	Intracranial pressure
IVH	Intraventricular hemorrhage
MCA	Middle cerebral artery
MRI	Magnetic resonance imaging
MTT	Mean transit time
PCA	Posterior cerebral artery
PLIC	Posterior limb of internal capsule
rCBF	Regional cerebral blood flow
rCBV	Regional cerebral blood volume
ROI	Region of interest
SAH	Subarachnoid hemorrhage
SDH	Subdural hematoma
SWAN	T2*-weighted angiography
TBI	Traumatic brain injury

Contents

1 Clinical and Prognostic Value of Neuroimaging in Traumatic Brain Injury 1
   1.1   TBI-Related Social and Economic Problems 1
   1.2   Neuroimaging in Assessment of Traumatic Brain Injury 3
   1.3   Classifications of Traumatic Brain Injury 4
   1.4   CT and MRI in TBI 5
         1.4.1   Conventional MRI Sequences in Diagnosis of TBI 6
         1.4.2   Advanced MRI Sequences in Diagnosis of TBI 7
         1.4.3   MRI Classification of TBI 8
         1.4.4   Other Neuroimaging Methods 8
   1.5   Diffusion-Tensor MRI and MR Tractography 9
   1.6   Cerebral Blood Flow Assessment 11
   1.7   Radiation Safety 14
   References 16

2 Clinical Evaluation and Neuroimaging Technologies 25
   2.1   Clinical Material 25
   2.2   Methods of Study 28
         2.2.1   Computed Tomography 28
         2.2.2   Magnetic Resonance Tomography 30
   2.3   Statistical Analysis 33
   References 33

3 Neuroimaging Classification of Traumatic Brain Injury 35
   3.1   CT and MRI Data Comparison 35
   3.2   MRI Classification of TBI 41
   3.3   Discussion 61
   References 66

**4   Dynamic Study of White Matter Fiber Tracts After
     Traumatic Brain Injury**..   69
     4.1   Quantitative Evaluation of Corpus Callosum
           and Corticospinal Tract Condition in the Acute Period of TBI.......   69
     4.2   Dynamic DT-MRI Study of Corpus Callosum
           and Corticospinal Tracts   74
     4.3   Discussion.. 102
     References.. 105

**5   Mapping of Cerebral Blood Flow in Focal and Diffuse
     Brain Injury**... 107
     5.1   Clinical Material 107
     5.2   Peculiarities of rCBF in Patients with Diffuse Axonal Injury......... 112
     5.3   Peculiarities of rCBF in Patients with DAI Combined
           with Focal Brain Contusions... 115
     5.4   Peculiarities of rCBF in Patients with Focal Brain Contusions....... 117
     5.5   Peculiarities of rCBF in the Contusion Areas................................ 119
     5.6   Study of rCBF in Subcortical Formations
           (Basal Ganglia and Thalami)... 119
     5.7   Discussion.. 119
     References.. 122

**6   Dynamics of Hemispheric and Brain Stem Regional
     Cerebral Blood Flow**... 125
     6.1   Clinical Material 125
     6.2   Dynamics of rCBF in Hemispheric Brain Structures 126
     6.3   Analysis of rCBF in the Brain Stem 138
     6.4   Dynamic Studies of rCBF in the Brain Stem................................. 141
     6.5   Discussion.. 146
     References.. 153

Index.. 155

Contents

1.1	TBI-Related Social and Economic Problems	1
1.2	Neuroimaging in Assessment of Traumatic Brain Injury	3
1.3	Classifications of Traumatic Brain Injury	4
1.4	CT and MRI in TBI	5
	1.4.1 Conventional MRI Sequences in Diagnosis of TBI	6
	1.4.2 Advanced MRI Sequences in Diagnosis of TBI	7
	1.4.3 MRI Classification of TBI	8
	1.4.4 Other Neuroimaging Methods	8
1.5	Diffusion-Tensor MRI and MR Tractography	9
1.6	Cerebral Blood Flow Assessment	11
1.7	Radiation Safety	14
References		16

1.1 TBI-Related Social and Economic Problems

More than 1.2 million people die every year with about 20–50 million getting non-fatal trauma in traffic accidents (Global status report on road safety 2009). Brain damage is the cause of death in approximately 60 % of all trauma-related fatalities (Potapov et al. 2010).

According to World Health Organization data, countries with low and middle income show higher road accident fatality level (21.5 and 19.5 per 100,000), while countries with high income demonstrate a lower level (10.3 per 100,000). More than 90 % fatalities as a result of traffic accidents are reported in countries with low and middle income (Global status report on road safety 2009). The leading causes of death and disability of population in various age groups worldwide are summarized in Table 1.1.

In Russia 600,000 people suffer from TBI every year including 50,000 fatal cases with the number of disabled exceeding two million (Potapov et al. 2003). Traffic accidents, falls, assaults, etc., are the leading causes of different severity of

Table 1.1 Leading causes of death by age worldwide, 2004 (shortened) (Global status report on road safety 2009)

Rank	0–4 years	5–14 years	15–29 years	30–44 years	45–69 years	70+	Total
1	Perinatal causes	Lower respiratory infections	Road traffic injuries	HIV/AIDS	Ischemic heart disease	Ischemic heart disease	Ischemic heart disease
2	Lower respiratory infections	Road traffic injuries	HIV/AIDS	Tuberculosis	Cerebrovascular disease	Cerebrovascular disease	Cerebrovascular disease
3	Diarrheal diseases	Malaria	Tuberculosis	Road traffic injuries	HIV/AIDS	Chronic obstructive pulmonary disease	Lower respiratory infections
4	Malaria	Drownings	Violence	Ischemic heart disease	Tuberculosis	Lower respiratory infections	Perinatal causes
5	Measles	Meningitis	Self-inflicted injuries	Self-inflicted injuries	Chronic obstructive pulmonary disease	Trachea, bronchus, lung cancer	Chronic obstructive pulmonary disease

Table 1.2   Leading causes of death, 2004 and 2030 compared (shortened) (Global status report on road safety 2009)

Total 2004			Total 2030		
Rank	Leading cause	%	Rank	Leading cause	%
1	Ischemic heart disease	12.2	1	Ischemic heart disease	14.2
2	Cerebrovascular disease	9.7	2	Cerebrovascular disease	12.1
3	Lower respiratory infections	7.0	3	Chronic obstructive pulmonary disease	8.6
4	Chronic obstructive pulmonary disease	5.1	4	Lower respiratory infections	3.8
5	Diarrheal disease	3.6	5	Road traffic injuries	3.6
6	HIV/AIDS	3.5	6	Trachea, bronchus, lung cancer	3.4
7	Tuberculosis	2.5	7	Diabetes mellitus	3.3
8	Trachea, bronchus, lung cancer	2.3	8	Hypertensive heart disease	2.1
9	Road traffic injuries	2.2	9	Stomach cancer	1.9
10	Prematurity and low birth weight	2.0	10	HIV/AIDS	1.8

brain trauma. TBI accounts for more than a half of trauma-related deaths, which is mostly common for traffic accidents (Teasdale et al. 1995; Marion et al. 1998).

By 2030, traffic accidents will be the 5th leading cause of death among all age groups worldwide (Global status report on road safety 2009) (Table 1.2).

Thus, motor vehicle-related neurotrauma and, first of all, head injury are the main causes of disability and mortality. The social significance of this problem makes us looking for new clinical methods of neurotrauma diagnosis and their introduction into clinical practice, as well as studying TBI pathogenesis and prognosis of outcome.

1.2   Neuroimaging in Assessment of Traumatic Brain Injury

In the 1970s, the introduction of computed tomography (CT) made it possible to visualize craniocerebral injury in vivo. Later appearance of magnetic resonance scanners with various sequences allowed better visualization of structural, metabolic, and functional aspects of the brain damage. Technological progress has made the basis for exponential improvement of the quality of imaging which is still ongoing. The beginning of the twenty-first century became the "golden" era for neuroimaging with its modern possibilities in studying structural and functional brain integrity, alongside with understanding brain functioning both in normal and pathological conditions.

When dealing with TBI, one should specify the mechanism of trauma and its extent and severity of cerebral and cranial damage. Timely identification of these factors allows prevention of numerous complications and irreversible changes. Different neuroimaging methods play the crucial role in the diagnostics of head injuries, their classification and extent, as well as distribution of patients for emergency surgery or intensive care. The recently developed CT and MRI modalities allow a better understanding of TBI pathophysiology, differentiating between primary and secondary brain damages. Primary brain injury occurs at the moment of direct impact, while secondary one evolves in minutes, hours, or days after the injury. Secondary factors can be prevented or treated depending on their timely and correct diagnosis, organization, and quality of the provided neurosurgical care (Gean 1994; Parizel et al. 2005; Potapov and Likhterman 2011).

1.3   Classifications of Traumatic Brain Injury

A widespread use of various imaging techniques has demonstrated that no universal method exists for studying different types of TBI and its consequences as well as evaluating a broad range of pathophysiological reactions of the brain at various posttraumatic periods. The clinical and morphological characteristics of the traumatic brain injury are used as the basis for development of the classification system for TBI. Attempts to classify TBI have been undertaken for a long time. In the pre-neuroimaging era, the specific emphasis was placed on their clinical manifestations, coma duration, posttraumatic amnesia, neurological and vegetative disorders, as well as on the results of postmortem studies of fatalities from TBI. The era of the computed tomography has permitted the development of classifications based on the lifetime morphological features of the brain injury. In particular, CT classifications were developed to identify various degrees of severity of focal contusions and diffuse injuries, intracranial hemorrhages, and hematomas (Gennarelli et al. 1982; Konovalov and Kornienko 1985; Marshall et al. 1991).

The following primary injuries are differentiated: focal contusions and lacerations, diffuse axonal injuries, primary brain stem injury, intracranial hemorrhages, etc. Secondary intracranial damages include delayed hematomas (epidural, subdural, intracerebral), cerebral blood flow and cerebrospinal fluid circulation disturbances as a result of subarachnoid or intraventricular hemorrhage, brain volume enlargement or brain swelling as a result of edema, hyperemia or venous congestion, intracranial hypertension, brain shift and herniation, etc. Secondary extracranial factors include arterial hypotension, hypoxemia, hypercapnia, anemia, etc. (Strich 1956; Gennarelli et al. 1982; Mendelow and Teasdale 1983; Povlishock 1986; Adams et al. 1989, 2000; Teasdale et al. 1995; Reilly and Bullock 2005; Potapov et al. 2011).

The following clinical forms of TBI can be identified: (1) brain concussion, (2) mild brain contusion, (3) moderate brain contusion, (4) severe brain contusion, (5) diffuse axonal injury, (6) brain compression, and (7) head compression.

An adequate staging and classification of TBI are obligatory conditions and the basis for studying pathological processes triggered by trauma, and developing effective methods for prevention and treatment of unfavorable consequences (Likhterman and Potapov 1998; Likhterman and Kasumova 2012; Potapov et al. 2011).

Smirnov (1949), the Russian morphologist and founder of the theory of the cerebral traumatic disease, defined it as a combination of etiology, pathological anatomy, pathophysiological mechanisms, its development, outcome, and complications.

Table 1.3 Diagnostic categories of types of abnormalities visualized on CT scanning (Marshall et al. 1991)

Category	Definition
Diffuse injury I (no visible pathology)	No visible intracranial pathology seen on CT scan
Diffuse injury II	Cisterns are present with midline shift 0–5 mm and/or lesion density present; no high-or mixed-density lesion > 25 cc May include bone fragments and foreign bodies
Diffuse injury III (swelling)	Cisterns compressed or absent with midline shift 0–5 mm; no high-or mixed-density lesion > 25 cc
Diffuse injury IV (shift)	Midline shift > 5 mm; no high-or mixed density lesion > 25 cc
Evacuated mass lesion	All lesions surgically evacuated
Non-evacuated mass lesion	High-or mixed-density lesion > 25 cc, not surgically evacuated

1.4   CT and MRI in TBI

The advantages of CT scanning, as a method of choice for primary examination of patients with TBI, include prompt visualization of acute intracranial hemorrhages with their location sites, mass effect, and edema and identification of size and configuration of the ventricular system and subarachnoid spaces, bone fractures, or presence of foreign bodies, etc. Additional positive quality of this technique is its availability, speed of scanning, and compatibility with other life-support equipment (Parizel et al. 2005; Daviz et al. 2008; Kornienko and Pronin 2009). Therefore, CT has the ability of identifying urgent surgical situations, especially for patients with severe trauma.

In 1982, Gennarelli et al. developed a CT and clinically relevant classification of severe head injury and subdivided patients by focal and diffuse types of lesions in addition to categorizing them by Glasgow Coma Scale and coma duration.

The classification proposed by Marshall et al. (1991) was mainly based on the results of primary CT scans of patients with severe TBI, signs of midline shift, and mesencephalic cistern compression. It comprised a four-category scale for diagnosis of diffuse injury and two categories for diagnosis of mass lesions with special emphasis being placed on their possible surgical removal (Table 1.3).

This classification has proved to be helpful for creating the data bank and performing clinical studies of efficacy of various treatment methods. It also helped to determine a significant correlation between four diagnostic categories of diffuse injury and mortality rate, as well as ICP increase. However, CT scanning does not always help to predict outcome, because in severe brain trauma CT may fail to identify some pathological changes. Diagnostic possibilities and sensitivity of CT imaging in less severe brain injuries and in those of nonhemorrhagic nature are less significant. It was shown that intracranial pathology was detected in 5 % of patients with mild trauma (Glasgow Coma Scale score of 15) and in 30 % of cases with GCS score of 13 or less (Borg et al. 2004; Parizel et al. 2005). Despite the fact that clinical symptoms may predict pathological changes on CT scans, particularly in severe or moderate traumatic brain injury, it is not absolutely true for mild trauma, especially in children.

In addition, CT has a low sensitivity for detecting small cerebral damage foci in mild head injury and especially those adjacent to the cranial base and roof bones, as well as diffuse axonal injury and brain stem damages. CT scanning is also considered as a relatively insensitive method for detecting acute hypoxic and ischemic cerebral changes, subacute and chronic hemorrhages, and differentiating types of brain edema (Daviz et al. 2008; Kornienko and Pronin 2009).

MRI is more sensitive than CT in detecting brain damage in spite of its difficult application in the acute period of TBI, much time spent for scanning, and sedation of patients with motor and psychomotor agitation. MRI has serious contraindications for patients with unstable hemodynamics, and the presence of metal implants or cardiac pacemakers makes the examination impossible. There is a necessity for using special non-magnetic monitoring and ventilation equipment during scanning time in patients with severe TBI (Huisman et al. 2003, 2004; Parizel et al. 2005; Kornienko and Pronin 2009).

It is well known that MRI is more sensitive than CT in detecting nonhemorrhagic lesions and, in particular, DAI and other types of TBI during the subacute and chronic stages. Conventional MRI sequences of T1, T2, T2-FLAIR, and T2* gradient echo demonstrate different changes in the brain structures – mass effect, cistern compression, small intraparenchymal hemorrhages, and accumulation of blood in the subarachnoid space. Hemosiderin-sensitive 2D T2* gradient echo is helpful in imaging of petechial, subacute, and chronic hemorrhages. Diffusion sequences improve detection of secondary acute infarctions in TBI. Up-to-date techniques are more sensitive to blood products (SWI, SWAN) and are useful in assessing cerebral perfusion (MR perfusion, ASL) and microstructural changes in the white matter tract integrity (diffusion-tensor MRI) and detecting brain activation areas (fMRI) (Gentry 1996; Sorensen et al. 1997; Liu et al. 1999; Huisman et al. 2003; Scheid et al. 2007; Daviz et al. 2008; Greenberg et al. 2009; Kornienko and Pronin 2009; Haacke et al. 2010).

1.4.1 Conventional MRI Sequences in Diagnosis of TBI

T1-weighted imaging is used to study anatomy of the brain. Processes that shorten T1 relaxation time result in the increased MR signal on T1 images, as, for instance, in hemorrhages with methemoglobin.

T2-weighted imaging is used to detect pathology with high water content in tissues, especially with edematous tissues, and is sensitive to deoxyhemoglobin and hemosiderin.

T2-FLAIR is described as a sequence of suppressed MR signal from the CSF and accentuated pathology revealed on T2 FSE sequences, especially with the abnormality being located in the cortical and periventricular regions, as well as diffuse axonal injury (Haacke et al. 2010). This impulse sequence also allows an accurate visualization of acute subarachnoid hemorrhages and has an equal or even higher sensitivity than CT (Campball and Zimmerman 1998; Parizel et al. 2005).

T2* gradient echo sequences are used for detection of small hemorrhages because of their high sensitivity to magnetic susceptibility effects. At the same time, small and petechial hemorrhages may be identified in the acute posttraumatic period, as well as in months and even years after trauma, when gradient echo sequences allow visualization of hypointense hemosiderin deposits after diffuse axonal injury (Parizel et al. 1998, 2001, 2005, Lin et al. 2001; Scheid et al. 2003).

1.4.2   Advanced MRI Sequences in Diagnosis of TBI

SWI (susceptibility-weighted imaging) and SWAN (T2 star-weighted angiography) are modern T2* sequence modifications and actually are 3D gradient echo with a high spatial resolution and flow compensation; they are especially sensitive to blood products in hemorrhages and deoxyhemoglobin in the venous blood (Reichenbach et al. 1997; Haacke et al. 2010; Pronin et al. 2011). SWI has proved to be more sensitive than 2D T2* GRE in diffuse axonal injury (Tong et al. 2004; Babikian et al. 2005; Haacke et al. 2010).

DWI – diffusion-weighted imaging – is sensitive to the motion of water molecules (hydrogen protons) in tissues; it allows a better understanding of brain physiology, with some of its aspects being impossible to study when using other sequences. DWI and apparent diffusion coefficient (ADC) obtained on maps are used in differential diagnosis of cytotoxic and vasogenic edema as a result of brain injury or ischemia (Kawamata et al. 2000; Huisman et al. 2003; Haacke et al. 2010). ADC reduction suggests presence of a cytotoxic (intracellular) edema, while its increase indicates development of a vasogenic (extracellular) edema. DWI plays the crucial role in detection of acute stroke and diffuse axonal injury (Liu et al. 1999; Haacke et al. 2010).

1H MR spectroscopy allows identification of various metabolites in the brain in vivo reflecting changes in both biochemical processes and structural damage of cells. Brain injury induces changes in N-acetylaspartate (NAA) (a neuronal biomarker), the decrease of which in pathology foci is indicative of its primary damage, while decrease in NAA in normally appearing brain areas may be indicative of DAI and Wallerian degeneration (Cecil et al. 1998a, b; Friedman et al. 1999; Brooks et al. 2000; Garnett et al. 2000, 2001; Portella et al. 2000; Yoon et al. 2005; Babikian et al. 2006; Holshouser et al. 2006; Shutter et al. 2006; Haacke et al. 2010). An increase in choline (Cho) levels (a marker for membrane disruption, synthesis, or repair) can be detected in the white matter and is associated with myelin damage (Ross et al. 1998; Haacke et al. 2010). Presence of lactate (Lac) (a result of anaerobic glycolysis) is indicative of a hypoxic/ischemic injury. Currently, two methods are used in proton MR spectroscopy – single- and multi-voxel modes. In single-voxel MR spectroscopy, only one region (voxel) of the brain is selected for the analysis. By analyzing frequencies of the signal registered from the voxel, the distribution of metabolite peaks is obtained by the chemical shift scale. In multi-voxel MR spectroscopy, MR spectra are obtained for several voxels simultaneously. That allows comparing spectra of different areas in the studied zone, as well as obtaining

Table 1.4 Group of abnormalities visualized on MRI (Firsching et al. 2001)

Diagnostic groups of lesions based on MRI after severe head injury	
Supratentorial injuries only	Grade I
Brain stem lesions with or without supratentorial lesions	Grade II, unilateral lesion of the brain stem at any levels ± I
	Grade III, bilateral lesion of the mesencephalon ± I–II
	Grade IV, bilateral pontine lesion ± I–III

parametric maps. The concentration of particular metabolites on these maps is marked by color, and thus it is possible to visualize the metabolite distribution in the brain (Kornienko and Pronin 2009).

1.4.3   MRI Classification of TBI

Based on the use of routine T1 and T2 MRI sequences and analysis of the data obtained from patients in the acute period of severe TBI, Firsching et al. (2001) proposed their classification of severe TBI (Table 1.4). According to the authors, an accurate location of lesion foci in the brain stem (primary or secondary) plays the crucial role in prognosis of TBI outcome.

At the same time, classification by Firsching et al. (2001) of the brain stem damage level was based on the results of routine MRI sequences and did not consider the mechanism of brain trauma and its severity and localization of supratentorial injuries. Mannion et al. (2007) studied 46 patients with acute severe TBI by using the following sequences: T2 MRI, proton density, FLAIR, and gradient echo imaging. The authors classified all patients into three groups based on the mechanism of brain stem injury: (1) brain stem lesions caused by DAI, (2) brain stem lesions as a result of supratentorial herniation, and (3) isolated brain stem lesions with small cortical contusions. It was shown that all patients in first and second groups showed unfavorable outcome in 6 months after trauma, while only two patients with isolated brain stem lesions had favorable outcome. Of 33 patients with supratentorial lesions, only 18 had unfavorable outcome. Despite an evidently significant relationship existing between brain stem lesions and unfavorable outcome, the authors have concluded that brain stem injury is not an absolute indicator of unfavorable outcomes. The role of MRI scanning in assessing the prognosis after severe and moderate TBI was also analyzed in studies of Kornienko and Pronin (2009), Lagares et al. (2009), and Hilario et al. (2012).

1.4.4   Other Neuroimaging Methods

SPECT, PET, xenon-enhanced CT, and fMRI are used in clinical practice when assessing cognitive and neuropsychological changes in patients with traumatic brain injury (Jacobs et al. 1994, 1996; Abdel-Dayem et al. 1998; Berrouschot et al. 1998; Weckesser and Schober 1999; Hofman et al. 2001; Warwick 2004;

Devous 2005; Daviz et al. 2008). These methods allow a qualitative assessment of cerebral perfusion that cannot be established with routine CT and MRI studies. The single-photon emission computer tomography (SPECT) reflects the brain perfusion only. Unlike SPECT, positron emission tomography (PET) has higher spatial resolution capabilities, which allows mapping of metabolism parameters in addition to the quantitative evaluation of the blood flow (Cikrit et al. 1997, 1999; Buttler et al. 1998; Wintermark et al. 2001a, b; Chen et al. 2004; Wu et al. 2004; Vespa et al. 2005; Wintermark et al. 2005; Catala-Temprano et al. 2007; Haacke et al. 2010). SPECT and PET in combination with CT or MRI are the most perspective ones in this regard. However, the main drawbacks of PET and SPECT are the necessity of using radiotracer, high cost, and insufficient availability in clinical settings.

Functional MRI (fMRI) is described as brain activation mapping based on hemodynamic response in the increased neuronal cortical activity as a response to the special motor, sensor, and other stimulation tasks (Kornienko and Pronin 2009). This method is used for studying various groups of patients with brain injury, yet it has not been introduced into routine clinical examinations of TBI. Functional MRI uses an echo-planar imaging approach and evaluates changes in the BOLD (blood oxygen level dependent) signal (Hattori et al. 2004; Strangman et al. 2005; Haacke et al. 2010). An increase in neuronal activity results in increase of blood flow, thus raising the local blood oxygenation levels (McAllister et al. 1999, 2006; Logothesis et al. 2001; Karunanayaka et al. 2007; Newsome et al. 2008; Strangman et al. 2009; Haacke et al. 2010). Functional MRI signal in brain injury can be modified as a result of change or combinations of changes of neuronal activity as well as regulation of the blood flow. Patients who are unable to perform special tests and tasks during fMRI cannot take part in these studies. The resting-state fMRI provides a new opportunity to study spontaneous fluctuations in the BOLD signal in TBI patients. This approach is an option to study patients with TBI of different severity ranging from concussion to vegetative state (Greicius et al. 2003; Nagai et al. 2004; Fox et al. 2005; Fox and Raichle 2007; Owen et al. 2006; Vincent et al. 2007; Haacke et al. 2010). However, the need for immobilization and sedation of patients with psychomotor agitation, seizures, or comatose state restricts the use of fMRI in TBI.

1.5 Diffusion-Tensor MRI and MR Tractography

Diffuse axonal injury (DAI) is one of the leading causes of morbidity and mortality in TBI patients. The anatomical structures that are most often injured in DAI are subcortical white matter, corpus callosum, dorsolateral regions of the midbrain, and subcortical formations (Strich 1956; Adams et al. 1982; Gennarelli et al. 1982, 1986; Gentry et al. 1988; Gean 1994; Murray et al. 1996; Povlishock and Stone 2001; Reilly and Bullock 2005).

Microscopic morphological studies demonstrated axonal damage in the form of axonal retraction balls already in 12 h following trauma. These balls are visible when being stained with silver impregnation (Kasumova 1998; Kasumova 1991) or by immunocytochemical method (Gentleman et al. 1993; Sheriff et al. 1994). In addition to the partial axonal damage, their subsequent condition depends on the degree of expression of secondary reactions – hemorrhages, edema, local perfusion changes, and various cascades of biochemical reactions (Gennarelli et al. 1986; Adams et al. 1989; Maxwell et al. 1997; Povlishock and Katz 2005).

Until recently, there has been no accurate method for in vivo diagnosis of prevalence and severity of DAI because CT and routine MRI poorly differentiate this type of injuries (Gentry et al. 1988; Kelly et al. 1988). CT findings characterized by petechial hemorrhages in the corpus callosum, white gray matter junction, and brain stem, more often the midbrain, could be seen only in 10 % of patients with severe DAI (Blumbergs et al. 1994, 1995; Xu et al. 2007). Delayed CT scans are often relatively normal or characterized by diffuse brain atrophy with the enlargement of ventricles and subarachnoid spaces (Whyte and Rosental 1993; Diaz-Marchan et al. 1996). Thus, more sensitive diagnostic methods should be found and used for diffuse axonal injury.

MRI, especially T2-FLAIR and T2* gradient echo, is much more sensitive for the accurate diagnosis and prognosis of TBI outcome depending on the level of hemispheric and brain stem damage (Firsching et al. 2001; Mannion et al. 2007). It was shown that the diffusion-weighted MRI (DWI) could reveal damages not visible even on T2, T2*, and T2-FLAIR MRI (Huisman et al. 2003).

An application of *diffusion-tensor MRI (DT MRI)* as well as the retrieval of 3D images has opened up new possibilities for the qualitative and quantitative assessment of brain pathway damage. Thus, in a clinical setting, in vivo, visualization of DAI severity can be obtained (Liu et al. 1999; Arfanakis et al. 2002; Huisman et al. 2004; Wilde et al. 2006; Benson et al. 2007; Kim et al. 2008; Zakharova et al. 2007, 2008, 2009, 2010a, b; Zakharova 2013).

DTI evaluates diffusion characteristics of water molecules in the region of interest as well as directional dependence of water diffusion (anisotropy) and, thus, provides information about the degree of white matter tract integrity (Melhem et al. 2000; Prefferbaum et al. 2000; Papadakis et al. 2002; Pronin et al. 2008). Diffusion anisotropy in different regions of the white matter is not uniform; it reveals differences in myelinization of fiber tracts, their diameter and orientation (Pierpaoli et al. 1996). Pathological processes that modify the white matter microstructure such as fiber disruption and separation, breakdown of myelin, neuronal swelling, and an increase or decrease of extracellular space have an impact on diffusion and anisotropy parameters (Ducreux et al. 2005; Povlishock and Katz 2005; Wilde et al. 2006; Grinberg et al. 2011).

The most commonly used quantitative values in the assessment of DWI and DTI are the apparent diffusion coefficient (ADC) and fractional anisotropy (FA), respectively (Basser and Pierpaoli 1996; Basser and Pierpaoli 1998). DTI studies in patients with head injuries have shown that FA is reduced in the first week after injury, despite of no changes in the white matter observed on CT or routine MRI (Arfanakis et al. 2002; Huisman et al. 2004). Reduced FA in cases with DAI was found in the anterior and posterior regions of the corpus callosum, posterior limb of the internal capsule and in the external capsule. Similar data were obtained in a study with a whole-brain white matter analysis of DTI data (Inglese et al. 2005; Benson et al. 2007).

It has been found that changes in diffusion-tensor parameters reflect degeneration of axons and myelin sheath leading to their atrophy. This process takes months and even years following DAI (van der Knaap 2005; Xu et al. 2007; Rutgers et al. 2008; Sidaros et al. 2008).

Individual observations of structural degeneration of corpus callosum fibers and fornix conducted at different time intervals following head injuries as well as varying severity have been described and visualized by MR tractography (Naganawa et al. 2004; Voss et al. 2006; Sugiyama et al. 2009). The commissural and projection pathways were chosen for a three-dimensional reconstruction in publications of various authors. It was based on the fact that the corpus callosum was easily distinguished with DTI on the midsagittal level by using colored fractional anisotropy mapping, while corticospinal tracts had a distinct unidirectionality. Other fiber tracts were more difficult to isolate especially on condition of high frequency and reproduction (Naganawa et al. 2004; Xu et al. 2007)

1.6   Cerebral Blood Flow Assessment

Brain perfusion disorders are the most common pathophysiological phenomena in TBI that is why studying cerebral hemodynamics is essential both for understanding pathogenic mechanisms of the traumatic brain disease and for developing treatment tactics and prognostic models (Meier and Zierler 1954; Contoni 1960; Fisher 1961; Reivich et al. 1961; Nariai et al. 1995, 1998; Mirzai and Saami 2000; Derdeyn et al. 2002). Research of rCBF disturbances became possible with the development of noninvasive methods of study, including positron emission tomography (PET), single-photon emission computer tomography (SPECT) (Madeau et al. 1995; Alexandrov et al. 1996; Launes et al. 1997; Davalos and Bennett 2002), xenon-enhanced CT (XeCT) (Ritter et al. 1999; Wintermark et al. 2001a), arterial spin labeling method (ASL) (Deibler et al. 2008a, b, c), as well as CT perfusion, MR perfusion (dynamic susceptibility contrast, DSC), and other methods (Shakhnovich and Shakhnovich 1996; Asenbaum and Baumgartner 2001; Garnett et al. 2001; Wintermark et al. 2005). CT perfusion method is the most available technique which is routinely used in diagnosis of acute stroke (Wintermark et al. 2008; Haacke et al. 2010), as well as in studying neoangiogenesis in patients with brain tumors (Covarrubias et al. 2004; Pronin et al. 2005; Kornienko and Pronin 2009; Haacke et al. 2010).

Xenon is a stable isotope and as a contrast material is easily diffused across the intact blood-brain barrier (Latchaw et al. 1987, 2003; Good et al. 1992). Xenon-enhanced CT is more commonly used in cerebrovascular diseases and rarely in TBI (Ritter et al. 1999; Wintermark et al. 2001b). This method provides an accurate quantitative cerebral blood flow evaluation, multilevel examination of the brain with an option of a 10 min interval examination repeat. The disadvantages of this method include a relatively long period of scanning and sensitivity to motion artifacts (Wintermark et al. 2005).

MR perfusion (dynamic susceptibility-weighted bolus-tracking MRI) method is based on the decrease of T2 or T2* relaxation times during the first passage of a contrast agent through the capillary network (Rosen et al. 1991; Ostergaard et al. 1996; Pronin et al. 2000; Grandin 2003; Kornienko and Pronin 2009). The advantages of this method are absence of ionizing radiation and allergic reactions to the contrast substance (gadolinium); however, its use is limited for cases of claustrophobia, presence of metal implants, etc. Similar to other methods, MR perfusion establishes the following parameters – MTT, CBV, CBF, and time to peak of contrast substance concentration (TTP). These parameters provide semiquantitative assessment of cerebral hemodynamics with calculation of the ratio or differences between the values obtained in a pathological area and similar area of the contralateral side, considered as reference normal values. It is important to note that no standardized interpretation has been proposed for such parameter maps (Wintermark et al. 2005). MR perfusion is usually used for diagnosis of acute stroke, chronic cerebrovascular diseases, and tumors (Sorensen et al. 1999; Sorensen and Reimer 2000; Pronin et al. 2000; Wintermark et al. 2005; Haacke et al. 2010). This method of CBF study is used in combination with anatomical MR images, DWI, MR spectroscopy, etc. At the same time, MR perfusion has significant limitations when being used for patients in severe conditions, including those in the acute period of TBI.

The arterial spin labeling (ASL) method is based on the proximal labeling of water protons with the preliminary saturation. The "labeled" spins enter (with blood flow) the vascular brain bloodstream and are responsible for decrease of MR signal from microvascular structures on dynamic MRI series. The second series is registered without preliminary saturation (in the absence of saturating radio frequency pulse), and the regional blood flow is calculated on the difference between these two series (Wintermark et al. 2005; Kornienko and Pronin 2009). There are two main ASL methods – pulsed and continuous techniques. No contrast media are needed, since endogenous water is used as a tracer. This method allows obtaining quantitative parameters of rCBF, which are accurate for the gray matter of the brain. However, different ASL models may either overestimate or underestimate blood flow in the white matter. Quantitative ASL perfusion maps produce approximately 10 % of changes during repeated scanning in the same subject. The difference between labeled and control acquisition signals is approximately 1 %; therefore, ASL perfusion monitoring requires a very high signal-to-noise ratio. Since the signal difference is low, the ASL cannot evaluate accurately blood flow maps below 10 ml/100 g/min. On the other hand, as the blood flow increases (in excess of 150 ml/100 g/min), this method may underestimate blood flow (Barbier et al. 2001; Wintermark et al. 2005; Petersen et al. 2006). Until recently, the ASL method has not been widely available in clinical practice. However, there are reports on its use in acute and chronic cerebrovascular pathologies, as well as in epilepsy and brain tumors (Wintermark et al. 2005; Petersen et al. 2006). The advantages of this method are absence of ionizing radiation and its noninvasiveness. The disadvantages of the method include rCBF underestimation in arterial and venous bypass areas, inclusion of the collateral blood flow, and limitations typical for any MRI study.

Each of the listed methods of the blood flow study has its advantages and disadvantages in various clinical settings.

It has passed over 50 years since Giliam and Janny (1951) and Lundberg (1960) described for the first time the method of continuous monitoring of intraventricular pressure. Today the intracranial pressure (ICP) monitoring is included into the guidelines for the management of severe traumatic brain injury based on the principles of evidence-based medicine (Bullock et al. 1996, 2000; Aarabi et al. 2001; Verweij et al. 2001; Potapov et al. 2003; Bratton et al. 2007). Direct measurements of arterial blood pressure and intracranial pressure (ICP) with a continuous assessment of cerebral perfusion pressure (CPP) form a mandatory component for modern neurological intensive care assessment and make the basis for an adequate support of the cerebral perfusion in patients with severe TBI (Lassen and Christenson 1976; Kornienko 1980; Bruce et al. 1981; Mendelow and Teasdale 1983; Glazman ct al. 1988, Potapov 1989; Ritter et al. 1999; Potapov et al. 2003; Reilly and Bullock 2005).

At the same time, CPP monitoring does not allow assessing the real status of tissue perfusion in different vascular regions, damage foci, perifocal area, etc.

CT perfusion is a relatively new minimally invasive method of visualization and quantitative mapping of rCBF that may be used in patients with various neurosurgical pathologies (Wintermark et al. 2001a, b, 2004a, b, 2005; Pronin et al. 2002, 2005; Kornienko and Pronin 2009). The advantage of the perfusion method is its short duration of CT study with further post-processing at workstation. The quantitative evaluation of the parameters of cerebral blood flow (rCBF), cerebral blood volume (rCBV), and mean transit time (MTT) in regions of interest (ROI) can be performed in the main vascular regions of the anterior, middle, and posterior cerebral arteries (Kudo et al. 2003; Wintermark et al. 2004a, b; Zakharova et al. 2006), as well as in minor areas of the white and gray matter (Schaefer et al. 2006; Pronin et al. 2007). It has been shown that rCBF parameters obtained by CT perfusion are quite similar to those of xenon-enhanced CT, positron emission tomography, and other methods (Kety and Schmidt 1948; Obrist et al. 1967; Kondakov 1976; Lassen and Christenson 1976; Potapov et al. 1978, 1979; Axel 1980; Kryvoshapkin 1982; Gaydar 1983, 1990; Glazman et al. 1988; Kondakov et al. 2001; Wintermark et al. 2001b; Kudo et al. 2003; Haacke et al. 2010).

CT perfusion can be used as a useful tool for a quick simple identification of ischemia in the acute stage of subarachnoid hemorrhage. It also may have a prognostic value and be useful for intracranial pressure management in patients with TBI (Wintermark et al. 2004a). A wide availability of CT as a part of emergency care departments and its short scanning time make it an ideal method for investigation of patients requiring urgent treatment, especially those with stroke (Wintermark et al. 2005). CT perfusion is an effective accurate quantitative method; however, it has a limited spatial coverage. Its other disadvantages are an ionizing radiation and usage of iodinated contrast material.

The first reports on the use of CT perfusion in cases of TBI have appeared only recently (Wintermark et al. 2004b; Zakharova et al. 2006). Based on the research results, Wintermark et al. (2004b) concluded that CT perfusion provided additional

Table 1.5 Relative radiation level designation (Daviz et al. 2008)

Relative radiation level	Effective dose, estimate range
None	0
Minimal	<0.1 mSv
Low	0.1–1 mSv
Medium	1–10 mSv
High	10–100 mSv

information to the conventional CT in traumatic brain injury. They studied changes in rCBF both in focal and diffuse brain injuries. It was shown that normal brain perfusion and hyperemia were associated with a favorable outcome, whereas oligemia and ischemia were associated with an unfavorable outcome. Local changes in perfusion may be observed in cerebral contusions with higher sensitivity when compared with admission unenhanced cerebral CT (Wintermark et al. 2004b, 2006; Soustiel et al. 2008; Haacke et al. 2010). In DAI, the statistically significant correlation was established between the data obtained by invasive methods of studying cerebral perfusion pressure (CPP) and noninvasive measurements in CT perfusion; and zones of blood flow pathology were identified (Belanger et al. 2007). CT perfusion provides information about cerebral autoregulation and its disturbances in a real-time state, while ICP monitoring and data of CPP are continuous processes. However, in aggressive treatment, ICP and arterial blood pressure can be normalized unlike regional cerebral perfusion (Chieregato et al. 2004). When comparing CPP data to the results of noninvasive methods like transcranial cerebral oximetry, CT perfusion is more useful in identification of blood flow heterogeneity in cerebral tissues (Wintermark et al. 2005). It is no doubt that CT perfusion is reported to be more sensitive in identifying focal contusions – up to 87.5 % (Wintermark et al. 2004b). Similar results were obtained when using other methods of study like SPECT and PET (Abdel-Dayem et al. 1987; Gray et al. 1992; Newton et al. 1992; Nedd et al. 1993; Bavetts et al. 1994) and MR perfusion (Tong et al. 2003). Blood flow values within cerebral contusions in CT perfusion are in agreement with the data obtained by other methods like xenon-enhanced CT (Hoelper et al. 2000; Wintermark et al. 2004b).

The main disadvantages of this method are the need for a short-term immobilization of patients (lasting a few minutes) and use of ionizing radiation and iodinated contrast medium, which always should be taken into consideration when multiple radiologic studies are required (Wintermark et al. 2000; Wintermark 2010).

1.7   Radiation Safety

Potentially unfavorable radiation effect is considered one of the most important factors for choosing this or that method of neuroimaging. So, a wide range of radiation exposure exists associated with various diagnostic procedures, and relative radiation level indicators must be included in every study. These levels are based on the effective dose which is a radiation dose quantity that is used to estimate patient total radiation risk associated with imaging procedures (Daviz et al. 2008) (Table 1.5).

Different levels of the effective absorbed dose are used in CBF study; for instance, in PET this dose is 0.5–2 mSv; in SPECT, 3.5–12 mSv; xenon CT, 3.5–10 mSv; and CT perfusion, 2–3 mSv (Wintermark et al. 2005). According to the FDA studies of 200 patients over the period of 18 months, an incorrect use of CT scanning protocols resulted in an eightfold excess of the expected radiation level (Wintermark 2010). The influence of such overexposure was significant: 40 % of patients lost patches of hair as a result of overdoses. One of the patients from the published cases of radiation overexposure underwent four studies of 120 κVp CT perfusion with CT angiograms and two conventional digital subtraction angiograms over a 2-week period (Imanishi et al. 2005). All medical institutions, especially neurological intensive care units where patients may need CT, CT AG, CT perfusion, and fluoroscopic examination practically simultaneously, should perform minimal multiple dynamic studies with the use of ionizing radiation (Mullins et al. 2004; Loftus et al. 2009). In such situations the quality of CT protocols and selection of scan parameters should play the crucial role. CT perfusion must be performed at 80 κVp and at no more than 200 mA (Wintermark et al. 2000). When using these parameters, an effective radiation dose of a single-slab CT perfusion study must be close to the dose received in the unenhanced head CT, i.e., 2–3 mSv (Konstas et al. 2009). The complete study protocol in CT perfusion includes unenhanced and post-contrast head CT and CT perfusion. Not every scan sequence can be used for every patient; the indications for studies must be clearly defined (Wintermark 2010).

Despite the availability of a large number of neuroimaging methods, each method has certain advantages and disadvantages for patients with TBI. Therefore, no optimal indications for using this or that method of neuroimaging have been developed for traumatic brain injury. Many questions remain in the series of clinical reports with these methods used (CT and MRI, in particular). There is an actual need for further study of relationships between severity, localization, and level of hemispheric and brain stem damages based on the data of clinical and MRI correlations. It is still unclear what localization and severity of damage not only to the brain stem but also to the thalamus, basal ganglia, corpus callosum, and other structures may cause various conscious disturbances in patients with different head injury severity and different length of coma.

Until recently, no dynamic assessments of the white matter fiber tracts as well as three-dimensional reconstruction of both the corpus callosum and corticospinal tracts in severe DAI have been available. The degree of fiber tract disruption in this type of brain injury resulting in serious disturbance of consciousness, mental disintegration, and sensory and motor function disorders is still unclear. Therefore, it is important to use DT-MRI in order to provide improved diagnosis and outcome prognosis in severe DAI.

At the same time, critical changes of rCBF values in focal contusions and perifocal areas (based on CT perfusion data) remain unclear. Besides, the role of regional hyperemia has not been thoroughly studied in cases of focal or diffuse injuries, after removal of intracranial hematomas and decompressive craniectomy. Until recently, no research has been undertaken to identify specific features of rCBF in the brain stem based on dynamic CT studies in the acute period of TBI.

The potential role of CT perfusion with its influence on choice of the treatment tactics in patients with TBI requires further detailed analysis. It is clear that rCBF values in hemispheric and brain stem structures must be considered during the treatment process when using different methods of ICP decrease and CPP maintenance.

Therefore, the study of structural and hemodynamic brain changes in severe traumatic brain injury using dynamic clinical, CT, and MRI studies remains very important.

References

Aarabi B, Alden T, Chesnut R et al (2001) Management and prognosis of penetrating brain injury. J Trauma 51:1–86

Abdel-Dayem H, Sadek H, Kouris K et al (1987) Changes in cerebral perfusion after acute head injury: comparison of CT with Tc-99m-HMPAO-SPECT. Radiology 165:221–226

Abdel-Dayem H, Abu-Judeh H, Kumar M et al (1998) SPECT brain perfusion abnormalities in mild or moderate traumatic brain injury. Clin Nucl Med 23:309–317

Adams J, Graham D, Murray L, Scott G (1982) Diffuse axonal injury due to nonmissile head injury in humans: an analysis of 45 cases. Ann Neurol 12:557–563

Adams J, Doyle D, Ford I et al (1989) Diffuse axonal injury in head injury: definition, diagnosis and grading. Histopathology 15:49–59

Adams JH et al (2000) The neuropathology of the vegetative state after acute insult. Brain 123: 1327–1338

Alexandrov A, Ehrlich L, Blandin C et al (1996) Simple visual analysis of brain perfusion on HMPAO SPECT predicts early outcome in acute stroke. Stroke 27:1537–1542

Arfanakis K, Haughton V, Carew J et al (2002) Diffusion tensor MR imaging in diffuse axonal injury. AJNR Am J Neuroradiol 23:794–802

Asenbaum S, Baumgartner C (2001) Nuclear medicine in the preoperative evaluation of epilepsy. Nucl Med Commun 22:835–840

Axel L (1980) Cerebral blood flow determination by rapid-sequence computed tomography. Radiology 137:679–686

Babikian T, Freier M, Tong K et al (2005) Susceptibility weighted imaging: neuropsychologic outcome and pediatric head injury. Pediatr Neurol 33:184–194

Babikian T, Freier M, Ashwal S et al (2006) MR spectroscopy: predicting long-term neuropsychological outcome following pediatric TBI. J Magn Reson Imaging 24:801–811

Barbier EL, Silva AC, Kim SG, Koretsky AP (2001) Perfusion imaging using dynamic arterial spin labeling (DASL). Magn Reson Med 45:1021–1029

Basser P, Pierpaoli C (1996) Microstructural and physiological features of tissues elucidated by quantitative – diffusion-tensor MRI. J Magn Reson 111:209–219

Basser P, Pierpaoli C (1998) A simplified method to measure the diffusion tensor from seven MR images. J Magn Reson Med 39:928–934

Bavetts S, Nimmon C, White J et al (1994) A prospective study comparing SPECT with MRI and CT as prognostic indicators following severe closed head injury. Nucl Med Common 15:961–968

Belanger H, Vanderploeg R, Curtiss G et al (2007) Recent neuroimaging techniques in mild traumatic brain injury. J Neuropsychiatry Clin Neurosci 19:5–20

Benson R, Meda S, Vasudevan S et al (2007) Global white matter analysis of diffusion tensor images is predictive of injury severity in traumatic brain injury. J Neurotrauma 24:446–459

Berrouschot J, Barthel H, Hesse S et al (1998) Differentiation between transient ischemic attack and ischemic stroke within the first six hours after onset of symptoms by using 99m-Tc-ECD-SPECT. J Cereb Blood Flow Metab 18:921–929

Blumbergs P, Scott G, Manavis J et al (1994) Staining of amyloid precursor protein to study axonal damage in mild head injury. Lancet 344:1055–1056

Blumbergs P, Scott G, Manavis J et al (1995) Topography of axonal injury as defined by amyloid precursor protein and the sector scoring method in mild and severe closed head injury. J Neurotrauma 12:565–572

Borg J, Holm L, Cassidi JD et al (2004) Diagnostic procedures in mild traumatic brain injury: results of the WHO collaborating centre task force on mild traumatic brain injury. J Rehabil Med 43(Suppl):61–75

Bratton S, Bullock R, Chesnut R et al (2007) Guidelines for the management of severe traumatic brain injury. J Neurotrauma 24(7):55–58

Brooks W, Stidley C, Petropoulos H et al (2000) Metabolic and cognitive response to human traumatic brain injury: a quantitative proton magnetic resonance study. J Neurotrauma 17:629–640

Bruce D, Alavi A, Bilamut M et al (1981) Diffuse cerebral swelling following head injuries in children: the syndrome of malignant brain edema. J Neurosurg 54(1):170–178

Bullock R, Chesnut R, Clifton G et al (1996) Guidelines for the management of severe traumatic brain injury. J Neurotrauma 13(11):639

Bullock R, Chesnut R, Clifton G et al (2000) Guidelines for management of severe traumatic brain injury. J Neurotrauma 17:451–553

Buttler C, Costa D, Walker Z et al (1998) PET and SPECT imaging in the dementias. In: Murray I, Ell P (eds) Nuclear medicine in clinical diagnosis and treatment, 2nd edn. Churchill Livingstone, Edinburgh, pp 713–728

Campball BG, Zimmerman RD (1998) Emergency magnetic resonance of the brain. Top Magn Reson Imaging 9:208–227

Catala-Temprano A, Claret Teruel G, Cambra Lasaosa F et al (2007) Intracranial pressure and cerebral perfusion pressure as risk factors in children with traumatic brain injuries. J Neurosurg 106(Suppl):463–466

Cecil K, Hills E, Sandel M et al (1998a) Proton magnetic resonance spectroscopy foe detection of axonal injury in the splenium of the corpus callosum of brain-injured patients. J Neurosurg 88:795–801

Cecil K, Lenkinski R, Meaney D et al (1998b) High-field proton magnetic resonance spectroscopy of a swine model for axonal injury. J Neurochem 70:2038–2044

Chen S, Richards H, Smielewski P et al (2004) Relationship between flow-metabolism uncoupling and evolving axonal injury after experimental traumatic brain injury. J Cereb Blood Flow Metab 24:1025–1036

Chieregato A, Fainardi E, Servadei F et al (2004) Centrifugal distribution of regional cerebral blood flow and its time course in traumatic intracerebral hematomas. J Neurotrauma 21:655–666

Cikrit D, Dalsing M, Harting P et al (1997) Cerebral vascular reactivity assessed with acetazolamide single photon emission computer tomography scans before and after carotid endarterectomy. Am J Surg 174:193–197

Cikrit D, Dalsing M, Lalka S et al (1999) The value of acetazolamide single photon emission computed tomography scans in the preoperative evaluation of asymptomatic critical carotid stenosis. J Vasc Surg 30:599–605

Covarrubias D, Rosen B, Lev M (2004) Dynamic magnetic resonance perfusion imaging of brain tumors. Oncologist 9:528–537

Contoni L (1960) The vertebro-vertebral collateral circulation in obliteration of the subclavian artery at its origin. Minerva Chir 15:268–271

Davalos D, Bennett T (2002) A review of the use of single-photon emission computerized tomography as a diagnostic tool in mild traumatic brain injury. Appl Neuropsychol 9:92–105

Daviz P, Brunberg J, De La Paz R et al (2008) Expert panel on neurologic imaging. ACR Appropriateness Criteria ® head trauma. [Online publication]. Reston, American College of Radiology (ACR) Web site, 13 p

Deibler A, Pollock J, Kraft R et al (2008a) Arterial spin-labeling in routine clinical practice, part 1: technique and artifacts. AJNR Am J Neuroradiol 29(7):1228–1234

Deibler A, Pollock J, Kraft R et al (2008b) Arterial spin-labeling in routine clinical practice, part 2: hypoperfusion patterns. AJNR Am J Neuroradiol 29(7):1235–1241

Deibler A, Pollock J, Kraft R et al (2008c) Arterial spin-labeling in routine clinical practice, part 3: hyperperfusion patterns. AJNR Am J Neuroradiol 29(8):1428–1435

Derdeyn C, Videen T, Yundt K et al (2002) Variability of cerebral blood volume and oxygen extraction: stages of cerebral hemodynamic impairment revisited. Brain 125:595–607

Devous M (2005) Single-photon emission computed tomography in neurotherapeutics. NeuroRx 2:237–249

Diaz-Marchan P, Hayman L, Carrier D et al (1996) Computed tomography of closed injury. In: Narayan R, Wilburger J, Povlishock J (eds) Neurotrauma. McGraw-Hill, New York, pp 137–149

Ducreux D, Huynh I, Fillard P et al (2005) Brain MR diffusion tensor imaging and fibre tracking to differentiate between two diffuse axonal injuries. Neuroradiology 47:604–608

Firsching R, Woischneck D, Klein S et al (2001) Classification of severe head injury based on magnetic resonance imaging. Acta Neurochir 143:263–271

Fisher CM (1961) A new vascular syndrome: "the subclavian steal". New Engl J Med 265: 912–913

Fox M, Raichle M (2007) Spontaneous fluctuations in brain activity observed with functional magnetic resonance imaging. Nat Rev Neurosci 8:700–711

Fox M, Snyder A, Vincent J et al (2005) The human brain is intrinsically organized into dynamic, anticorrelated functional networks. Proc Natl Acad Sci U S A 102:9673–9678

Friedman S, Brooks W, Jung R et al (1999) Quantitative proton MRS predicts outcome after traumatic brain injury. Neurology 52:1384–1391

Garnett M, Blamire A, Corkill R et al (2000) Early proton magnetic resonance spectroscopy in normal-appearing brain correlates with outcome in patients following traumatic brain injury. Brain 123(Pt10):2046–2054

Garnett M, Corkill R, Blamire A et al (2001) Altered cellular metabolism following traumatic brain injury: a magnetic resonance spectroscopy study. J Neurotrauma 18:231–240

Gaydar B (1983) Diagnostic and prognostic value of cerebral vessels reactivity parameters in the acute stage of head injury. Dissertation, Military Medical Academy, Leningrad

Gaydar B (1990) Principles of optimization of cerebral hemodynamics in neurosurgical pathology of the brain (clinical and experimental study). Dissertation, Military Medical Academy, Leningrad

Gean AD (1994) White matter shearing injury and brainstem injury. In: Gean AD (ed) Imaging of head trauma. Raven, New York, pp 207–248

Gennarelli T, Thibault L, Adams J et al (1982) Diffuse axonal injury and traumatic coma in the primate. Ann Neurol 12:564–574

Gennarelli T, Adams J, Graham D (1986) Diffuse axonal injury – a new conceptual approach to an old problem. In: Baethman A et al (eds) Mechanism of secondary brain damage. Plenum, New York, pp 15–28

Gentleman S, Nash M, Sweeting C et al (1993) Beta-amyloid precursor protein (beta APP) as a marker for axonal injury after head injury. Neurosci Lett 160:139–144

Gentry L (1996) Head trauma. In: Atlas SW (ed) Magnetic resonance imaging of the brain and spine. Raven, New York, pp 611–647

Gentry L, Godersky J, Thompson B et al (1988) Prospective comparative study of intermediate-field MR and CT in the evaluation of closed head trauma. AJR Am J Roentgenol 150:673–682

Giliam J, Janny P (1951) Manomatric intracranienne continue: interet de la mathode et premiera resultatas. Rev Neurol 84(2):131–142

Glazman L, Potapov A, Tomas J (1988) Hemispheric cerebral blood flow in different types of traumatic brain injury. Zh Vopr Neurokhir im NNBurdenko 4:35–39

Global status report on road safety: time for action (2009) Geneva, World Health Organization. http://www.who.int/violence_injury_prevention/road_safety_status/2009

Good W, Gur D, Yonas H (1992) Technical aspects. In: Yonas H (ed) Cerebral blood flow measurement with stable xenon-enhanced computed tomography. Raven, New York, pp 4–15

Grandin CB (2003) Assessment of brain perfusion with MRI: methodology and application to acute stroke. Neuroradiology 45:755–766

Gray B, Ischise M, Chung D et al (1992) Technetium-99m-HMPAO SPECT in the evaluation of patients with remote history of traumatic brain injury: a comparison with x-ray computed tomography. J Nucl Med 33:52–58

Greenberg S, Vernooij M, Cordonnier C et al (2009) Cerebral microbleeds: a guide to detection and interpretation. Lancet Neurol 8:165–174

Greicius M, Krasnow B, Reiss A et al (2003) Functional connectivity in the resting brain: a network analysis of the default mode hypothesis. Proc Natl Acad Sci U S A 100:253–258

Grinberg F, Farrher E, Kaffanke J (2011) Non-Gaussian diffusion in human brain tissue at high b-factors as examined by a combined diffusion kurtosis and biexponential diffusion tensor analysis. Neuroimage 57:1087–1112

Haacke E, Duhaime A, Gean A et al (2010) Common data elements in radiologic imaging of traumatic brain injury. J MRI 32(3):516–543

Hattori N, Huang S, Wu H et al (2004) Acute changes in regional cerebral (18)F-FDG kinetics in patients with traumatic brain injury. J Nucl Med 45:775–783

Hilario A, Ramos A, Millan JM et al (2012) Severe traumatic head injury: prognostic value of brain stem injuries detected at MRI. AJNR Am J Neuroradiol 33:1925–1931

Hoelper B, Reinert M, Zauner A et al (2000) rCBF in hemorrhagic, non-hemorrhagic and mixed contusions after severe head injury and its effect on perilesional cerebral blood flow. Acta Neurochir Suppl 76:21–25

Hofman P, Stapert S, van Kroonenburgh M et al (2001) MR imaging, single-photon emission CT, and neurocognitive performance after mild traumatic brain injury. AJNR Am J Neuroradiol 22:441–449

Holshouser B, Tong K, Ashwal S et al (2006) Prospective longitudinal proton magnetic resonance spectroscopic imaging in adult traumatic brain injury. J Magn Reson Imaging 24:33–40

Huisman T, Sorensen A, Hergan K et al (2003) Diffusion-weighted imaging for the evaluation of diffuse axonal injury in closed head injury. J Comput Assist Tomogr 27:5–11

Huisman T, Schwamm L, Schaefer P et al (2004) Diffusion tensor imaging as potential biomarker of white matter injury in diffuse axonal injury. AJNR Am J Neuroradiol 25:370–376

Imanishi Y, Fukui A, Niimi H et al (2005) Radiation-induced temporary hair loss as a radiation damage only occurring in patients who had the combination of MDCT and DSA. Eur Radiol 15:41–46

Inglese M, Makani S, Johnson G et al (2005) Diffuse axonal injury in mild traumatic brain injury: a diffusion tensor imaging study. J Neurosurg 103:298–303

Jacobs A, Put E, Ingels M et al (1994) Prospective evaluation of technetium -99m-HMPAO SPECT in mild and moderate traumatic brain injury. J Nucl Med 35(6):942–947

Jacobs A, Put E, Ingels M et al (1996) One-year follow-up of technetium-99m-HMPAO SPECT in mild head injury. J Nucl Med 37:1605–1609

Karunanayaka P, Holland S, Yuan W et al (2007) Neural substrate differences in language networks and associated language-related behavioral impairments in children with TBI: a preliminary fMRI investigation. Neurorehabilitation 22:355–369

Kasumova A (1991) Dynamics of morphological changes in focal and diffuse brain injuries. In: Abstracts of all-USSR neurosurgical conference on trauma of the central nervous system, Odessa, 1991, pp 52–54

Kasumova S (1998) Pathologic anatomy of traumatic brain injury. In: Konovalov A, Likhterman L, Potapov A (eds) Clinical guidelines on traumatic brain injury, vol 1, Antidor, Moscow, p 169–229

Kawamata T, Katayama Y, Aoyama N et al (2000) Heterogenous mechanisms of early edema formation in cerebral contusion: diffusion MRI and ADC mapping study. Acta Neurochir Suppl 76:9–12

Kelly A, Zimmerman R, Snow R et al (1988) Head trauma: comparison of MR and CT – experience in 100 patients. AJNR Am J Neuroradiol 9:699–708

Kety SS, Schmidt CF (1948) The nitrous oxide method for the quantitative determination of cerebral blood flow in man: theory, procedure, and normal values. J Clin Invest 27:476–483

Kim J, Avants B, Patel S et al (2008) Structural consequences of diffuse traumatic brain injury: a large deformation tensor-based morphometry study. Neuroimage 39:1014–1026

Kondakov E (1976) Regional cerebral blood flow and pO2 in patients with severe brain contusion in the acute period. Dissertation, Polenov Neurosurgical institute, Leningrad

Kondakov E, Semenyutin V, Gaydar B (2001) Severe traumatic brain injury (functional and structural surroundings of the concussion zone and variants of surgery). Desyatka, St. Petersburg, pp 9–101

Konovalov A, Kornienko V (1985) Computed tomography in neurosurgery. Medicine, Moscow

Konstas A, Goldmakher G, Lee T et al (2009) Theoretic basis and technical implementations of CT perfusion in acute ischemic stroke, part 1: theoretic basis. AJNR Am J Neuroradiol 30: 662–668

Kornienko V (1980) Functional cerebral angiography in neurosurgical clinic. Medicine, Moscow

Kornienko V, Pronin I (eds) (2009) Diagnostic neuroradiology. Springer, Berlin/Heidelberg

Kryvoshapkin A (1982) Cerebral blood supply in the carotid and vertebral-basilar systems in traumatic brain injury. Dissertation, Novosibirsk medical institute

Kudo K et al (2003) Quantitative cerebral blood flow measurement with dynamic perfusion CT using the vascular-pixel elimination method: comparison with H_2O^{15} positron emission tomography. AJNR Am J Neuroradiol 24:419–426

Lagares A, Ramos A, Derez-Nunes A et al (2009) The role of MRI in assessing prognosis after severe and moderate head injury. Acta Neurochir 151:341–356

Lassen N, Christenson M (1976) Physiology of cerebral blood flow. Br J Anaesth 48:719–734

Latchaw R, Yonas H, Pentheny S et al (1987) Adverse reactions to xenon-enhanced CT cerebral blood flow determination. Radiology 163:251–254

Latchaw R, Yonas H, Hunter G et al (2003) Council on cardiovascular radiology of the American Heart Association. Guidelines and recommendations for perfusion imaging in cerebral ischemia. Stroke 34:1084–1104

Launes J, Siren J, Valanne L et al (1997) Unilateral hyperperfusion in brain-perfusion SPECT predicts poor prognosis in acute encephalitis. Neurology 48:1347–1351

Likhterman L, Kasumova S (2012) Periodization of the clinical course of TBI. In: Konovalov A et al (eds) Reconstructive and minimally invasive surgery of head injury sequelae. TA Alexeeva, Moscow, pp 47–54

Likhterman L, Potapov A (1998) Classification of the traumatic brain injury. In: Konovalov A, Likhterman L, Potapov A (eds) Clinical guidelines on traumatic brain injury, vol 1. Antidor, Moscow, pp 47–129

Lin D, Filippi C, Steever A, Zimmerman R (2001) Detection of intracranial hemorrhage: comparison between gradient-echo images and b(0) images obtained from diffusion-weighted echo-planar sequences. AJNR Am J Neuroradiol 22:1275–1281

Liu A, Maldjian J, Bagley L et al (1999) Traumatic brain injury: diffusion-weighted MR imaging findings. AJNR Am J Neuroradiol 20:1636–1641

Loftus M, Minkowitz S, Min R et al (2009) Reduction radiation exposure in aneurysmal subarachnoid hemorrhage. Radiological Society of North America annual meeting, Chicago, 2009

Logothetis N, Pauls J, Augath M et al (2001) Neurophysiological investigation of the basis of the fMRI signal. Nature 412:150–157

Lundberg N (1960) Continuous recording and control of ventricular fluid pressure in neurosurgical practice. Acta Psychiatr Scand 36(suppl149):1

Madeau J, Abdel-Dayem H, van Heertum R et al (1995) Head trauma: use of SPECT. J Neuroimaging 5(suppl 1):S53–S57

Mannion R, Cross J, Bradley P et al (2007) Mechanism-based MRI classification of traumatic brainstem injury and its relationship to outcome. J Neurotrauma 24:128–135

Marion D et al (1998) Head and spinal cord injury. Neurol Clin 16:485–502

Marshall L, Marshall S, Klauber M, Clark M (1991) A new classification of head injury based on computerized tomography. J Neurosurg 75:14–20

Maxwell W, Povlishock J, Graham D (1997) A mechanistic analysis of nondisruptive axonal injury. A review. J Neurotrauma 14:419–440

McAllister T, Saykin A, Flashman L et al (1999) Brain activation during working memory 1 month after mild traumatic brain injury: a functional MRI study. Neurology 53:1300–1308

McAllister T, Flashman L, McDonald B et al (2006) Mechanisms of working memory dysfunction after mild and moderate TBI: evidence from functional MRI and neurogenetics. J Neurotrauma 23:1450–1467

Meier P, Zierler K (1954) On the theory of the indicator-dilution method for measurement of blood flow and volume. J Appl Physiol 6:731–744

Melhem E, Itoh R, Jones L et al (2000) Diffusion tensor MR imaging of the brain: effect of diffusion weighting on trace and anisotropy measurements. AJNR Am J Neuroradiol 21:1813–1820

Mendelow A, Teasdale G (1983) Pathophysiology of head injuries. Br J Surg 70(11):641–650

Mirzai S, Saami M (2000) CBF determination in brain stem and cerebellar hemispheres. Keio J Med 49(Suppl 1):A45–A50

Mullins M, Lev M, Bove P et al (2004) Comparison of image quality between conventional and low-dose nonenhanced head CT. AJNR Am J Neuroradiol 25:533–538

Murray J, Gean A, Evans S (1996) Imaging of acute head injury. Semin ultrasound CT MR 17:185–205

Nagai Y et al (2004) Brain activity relating to the contingent negative variation: an fMRI investigation. Neuroimage 21:1232–1241

Naganawa S, Sato C, Ishihra S et al (2004) Serial evaluation of diffusion tensor brain fiber tracking in a patient with severe diffuse axonal injury. AJNR Am J Neuroradiol 25:1553–1556

Nariai T, Suzuki R, Hirakawa K et al (1995) Vascular reserve in chronic cerebral ischemia measured by the acetazolamide challenge test: comparison with positron emission tomography. AJNR Am J Neuroradiol 16:563–570

Nariai T, Senda M, Ishii K et al (1998) Posthyperventilatory steal response in chronic cerebral hemodynamic stress: a positron emission tomography study. Stroke 29:1281–1292

Nedd K, Stakianakis G, Ganz W et al (1993) 99mTc-HMPAO SPECT of the brain in mild to moderate traumatic brain injury patients compared with CT: a prospective study. Brain Inj 7:469–479

Newsome M, Steinberg J, Scheibel R et al (2008) Effects of traumatic brain injury on working memory-related brain activation in adolescents. Neuropsychology 22:419–425

Newton M, Greenwood R, Britton K et al (1992) A study comparing SPECT with CT and MRI after closed head injury. J Neurol Neurosurg Psychiatry 55:92–94

Obrist W, Thompson H, King C et al (1967) Determination of regional cerebral blood flow by inhalation of 133-Xenon. Circ Res 20:124–135

Ostergaard L, Weisskoff R, Chesler D et al (1996) High resolution measurement of cerebral blood flow using intravascular tracer bolus passages. Magn Reson Med 36:715–726

Owen AM et al (2006) Detecting awareness in the vegetative state. Science 313:1402

Papadakis N, Martin K, Mustafa M et al (2002) Study of the effect of CSF suppression on white matter diffusion anisotropy mapping of healthy human brain. Magn Reson Med 38:394–398

Parizel P, Ozsarlak O, Van Goethem J et al (1998) Imaging findings in diffuse axonal injury after closed head trauma. Eur Radiol 8:960–965

Parizel P, Makkat S, Van Miert E et al (2001) Intracranial hemorrhage: principles of CT and MRI interpretation. Eur Radiol 11:1770–1783

Parizel P, Van Goethem J, Ozsarlak O et al (2005) New developments in the neuroradiological diagnosis of craniocerebral trauma. Eur Radiol 15:569–581

Petersen E, Zimine I, Ho Y et al (2006) Non-invasive measurement of perfusion: a critical review of arterial spin labeling techniques. Br J Radiol 79:688–701

Pierpaoli C, Jezzard P, Basser P et al (1996) Diffusion tensor MR imaging of the human brain. Radiology 201:637–648

Portella G, Beaumont A, Corwin F et al (2000) Characterizing edema associated with cortical contusion and secondary insult using magnetic resonance spectroscopy. Acta Neurochir Suppl 76:273–275

Potapov A (1989) Pathogenesis and differentiated treatment of focal and diffuse brain injuries. Dissertation, Kiev neurosurgical institute

Potapov A, Likhterman L, Kravchuk A, Kornienko V, Zakharova N, Oshorov A, Filatova M (2010) Modern approaches to studying and treatment of traumatic brain injury. Annals clinical and experimental neurology 4(1):4–12

Potapov A, Likhterman L (2011) Management of severe traumatic brain injuries. In: Kalangu K, Kato Y, Dechambinoit G (eds) Essential practice of neurosurgery. WFNS. Asses Publishing Co Ltd, Japan, p 1460

Potapov A, Manevich A, Sirovsky E (1978) Mass-spectrometry in a complex study of life support systems of the brain after neurosurgical interventions. Anesteziol Reanimatol 1:22–25

Potapov A, Sirovsky E, Manevich A, Fedorov S (1979) Results of mass-spectrometric studies of oxygen, carbonic acid tension and cerebral blood flow in brain tissues of neurosurgical patients. Zh Vopr Neurokhir im NNBurdenko 1:20–26

Potapov A, Likhterman L, Zelman V, Kornienko V, Kravchuk A (eds) (2003) Evidence-based neurotraumatology. Andreeva TM, Moscow

Potapov A, Zakharova N, Pronin I et al (2011) Prognostic value of ICP, CPP and regional blood flow monitoring in diffuse and focal traumatic cerebral lesions. Vopr Neurochir 75(3):3–16

Povlishock J (1986) Traumatically induced axonal damage without concomitant change in focally related neuronal somata and dendrites. Acta Neuropathol 70:53–59

Povlishock J, Katz D (2005) Update of neuropathology and neurological recovery after traumatic brain injury. J Head Trauma Rehabil 20:76–94

Povlishock J, Stone J (2001) Traumatic axonal injury. In: Miller L, Hayes R (eds) Head trauma: basic, preclinical and clinical directions. Wiley-Liss, New York, pp 281–302

Prefferbaum A, Sullivan E, Hedehus M et al (2000) Age-related decline in brain white matter anisotropy measured with spatially corrected echo-planar diffusion tensor imaging. Magn Reson Med 44:259–268

Pronin I et al. (2000) Perfusion MRI (PWI) in differential diagnosis of brain neoplasms. In: Abstracts of the first symposium on CT and MRI brain perfusion imaging, Giessen, 6–8 Oct 2000

Pronin I, Fadeeva L, Rodionov P, Kornienko V (2002) CT perfusion in differential diagnosis of brain skull base tumors. In: Abstracts of XVIIth symposium neuroradiologicum, Paris, 18–24 Aug 2000, p 1S38

Pronin I et al (2005) Application of CT-perfusion in stereotactic biopsy for diffuse gliomas. In: Abstracts of nevsky neurological forum, St. Petersburg, 2005, p 189

Pronin I, Fadeeva L, Zakharova N, Dolgushin M, Kornienko V (2007) Perfusion CT: evaluation of cerebral blood flow in normal subject. Med Visualiz 3:8–12

Pronin I, Fadeeva L, Zakharova N et al (2008) Diffusion-tensor imaging and diffusion-tensor tractography. Ann Clin Exp Neurol 2(1):32–40

Pronin I, Turkin A, Dolgushin M et al (2011) Tissue contrast based on magnetic susceptibility: application in neuroradiology. Med Visualiz 3:75–84

Reichenbach J, Venkatesan R, Schillinger D et al (1997) Small vessels in the human brain: MR venography with deoxyhemoglobin as an intrinsic contrast agent. Radiology 204(56):36–50

Reilly P, Bullock R (2005) Head injury – pathophysiology and management, 2nd edn. Hodder Arnold, London

Reivich M, Holling H, Robert B et al (1961) Reversal of blood flow through the vertebral artery and its effect on cerebral circulation. New Engl J Med 265:878–885

Ritter A, Muizelaar J, Barnes T et al (1999) Brain stem blood flow, papillary response, and outcome in patients with severe head injuries. Neurosurgery 44(5):941–948

Rosen B, Belliveau J, Aronen H et al (1991) Susceptibility contrast imaging of cerebral blood volume: human experience. Magn Res Med 22:293–299

Ross B, Ernst T, Kreis R et al (1998) 1H MRS in acute traumatic brain injury. J Magn Reson Imaging 8:829–840

Rutgers D, Fillard P, Paradot G et al (2008) Diffusion tensor imaging characteristics of the corpus callosum in mild, moderate, and severe traumatic brain injury. AJNR Am J Neuroradiol 29:1730–1735

Schaefer P, Roccatagliata L, Ledezma C et al (2006) First-pass quantitative CT perfusion identifies thresholds for salvageable penumbra in acute stroke patients treated with intra-arterial therapy. AJNR Am J Neuroradiol 27:20–25

Scheid R, Preul C, Gruber O et al (2003) Diffuse axonal injury associated with chronic traumatic brain injury: evidence from T2*-weighted gradient-echo imaging at 3T. AJNR Am J Neuroradiol 24:1049–1056

Scheid R, Ott D, Roth H et al (2007) Comparative magnetic resonance imaging at 1.5 and 3.0 Tesla for the evaluation of traumatic microbleeds. J Neurotrauma 24:1811–1816

Shakhnovich A, Shakhnovich V (eds) (1996) Diagnostics of cerebral blood flow disturbances. Transcranial dopplerography. AST, Moscow

Sheriff F, Bridges L, Sivaloganathan S et al (1994) Early detection of axonal injury after human head trauma using immunocytochemistry for beta-amyloid precursor protein. Acta Neuropathol 87:55–62

Shutter L, Tong K, Lee A et al (2006) Prognostic role of proton magnetic resonance spectroscopy in acute traumatic brain injury. J Head Trauma Rehabil 21:334–349

Sidaros A, Engberg A, Sidaros K et al (2008) Diffusion tensor imaging during recovery from severe traumatic brain injury and relation to clinical outcome: a longitudinal study. Brain 131:559–572

Smirnov L (1949) Pathologic anatomy and pathogenesis of traumatic diseases of the nervous system. Academy of Medical Sciences of the USSR, Moscow

Sorensen A, Reimer P (2000) Cerebral MR Perfusion Imaging. Georg Thieme Verlag, Stuttgart NewYork

Sorensen A, Tievsky A, Ostergaard L et al (1997) Contrast agents in functional MR imaging. J Magn Reson Imaging 7:47–55

Sorensen A, Wu O, Copen W et al (1999) Human acute cerebral ischemia: detection of changes in water diffusion anisotropy by using MR imaging. Radiology 212:785–792

Soustiel J, Mahamid E, Goldsher D, Zaaroor M (2008) Perfusion CT for early assessment of traumatic cerebral contusion. Neuroradiology 50:189–196

Strangman G, O'Neil-Pirozzi T, Burke D et al (2005) Functional neuroimaging and cognitive rehabilitation for people with traumatic brain injury. Am J Phys Med Rehabil 84:62–75

Strangman G, Goldstein R, O'Neil-Pirozi T et al (2009) Neurophysiological alterations during strategy-based verbal learning in traumatic brain injury. Neurorehabil Neural Repair 23:226–236

Strich S (1956) Diffuse degeneration of the cerebral white matter in severe dementia following head injury. J Neurol Neurosurg Psychiatry 19:163–185

Sugiyama K, Kondo T, Oouchida Y et al (2009) Clinical utility of diffusion tensor imaging for evaluating patients with diffuse axonal injury and cognitive disorders in the chronic stage. J Neurotrauma 26:1879–1890

Teasdale G et al (1995) Head injury. J Neurol Neurosurg Psychiatry 58(5):526–539

Tong K, Ashwal S, Holshouser B et al (2003) Hemorrhagic shearing lesions in children and adolescents with posttraumatic diffuse axonal injury: improved detection and initial results. Radiology 227:332–339

Tong K, Ashwal S, Holshouser B et al (2004) Diffuse axonal injury in children: clinical correlation with hemorrhagic lesions. Ann Neurol 56:36–50

van der Knaap M (2005) Wallerian degeneration and myelin loss secondary to neuronal and axonal degeneration. In: van der Knaap M, Valk J (eds) Magnetic resonance of myelination and myelin disorders, 3rd edn. Springer, Heidelberg, pp 832–839

Verweij B, Muizelaar J, Vonas F et al (2001) Hyperacute measurement of intracranial pressure, cerebral perfusion pressure, jugular venous oxygen saturation, and laser Doppler flowmetry, before and during removal of traumatic acute subdural hematoma. J Neurosurg 95:569–572

Vespa P, Bergsneider M, Hattori N et al (2005) Metabolic crisis without brain ischemia is common after traumatic brain injury: a combined microdialysis and positron emission tomography study. J Cereb Blood Flow Metab 25:763–774

Vincent J, Patel G, Fox M et al (2007) Intrinsic functional architecture in the anaesthetized monkey brain. Nature 447:83–86

Voss H, Ulug A, Dyke J et al (2006) Possible axonal regrowth in late recovery from the minimally conscious state. J Clin Invest 116(7):2005–2011

Warwick J (2004) Imaging of brain function using SPECT. Metab Brain Dis 19:113–123

Weckesser M, Schober O (1999) Brain death revisited: utility confirmed for nuclear medicine. Eur J Nucl Med 26:1387–1391

Whyte J, Rosental M (1993) Rehabilitation of the patient with head injury. In: DeLisa JA (ed) Rehabilitation medicine: principles and practice. JBI Lippincott Company, Philadelphia, pp 825–860

Wilde E, Chu Z, Bigler E et al (2006) Diffusion tensor imaging in the corpus callosum in children after moderate to severe traumatic brain injury. J Neurotrauma 23:1412–1426

Wintermark M (2010) FDA investigates the safety of brain perfusion CT. AJNR Am J Neuroradiol 31:2–3

Wintermark M, Maeder P, Verdun F et al (2000) Using 80kVp versus 120 Kvp in perfusion CT measurement of regional cerebral blood flow. AJNR Am J Neuroradiol 21:1881–1884

Wintermark M, Maeder P, Thiran JP et al (2001a) Quantitative assessment of regional cerebral blood flow by perfusion CT studies at low injection rates: a critical review of the underlying theoretical models. Eur Radiol 11(7):1220–1230

Wintermark M, Thiran JP, Maeder P et al (2001b) Simultaneous measurements of regional cerebral blood flow by perfusion-CT and stable xenon-CT: a validation study. AJNR Am J Neuroradiol 22:905–914

Wintermark M, Chiolero R, van Melle G et al (2004a) Relationship between brain perfusion computed tomography variables and cerebral perfusion pressure in severe head trauma patients. Crit Care Med 32(7):1579–1587

Wintermark M, van Melle G, Schnyder P et al (2004b) Admission perfusion CT: prognostic value in patients with severe head trauma. Radiology 232:211–220

Wintermark M, Sesay M, Barbier E et al (2005) Comparative overview of brain perfusion imaging techniques. Stroke 36(9):83–99

Wintermark M, Chiolero R, van Melle G et al (2006) Cerebral vascular autoregulation assessed by perfusion-CT in severe head trauma patients. J Neuroradiol 33:27–37

Wintermark M, Albers G, Alexandrov A et al (2008) Acute stroke imaging research roadmap. AJNR Am J Neuroradiol 29:23–30

Wu H, Huang S, Hattori N et al (2004) Selective metabolic reduction in gray matter acutely following human traumatic brain injury. J Neurotrauma 21:149–161

Xu J, Rasmussen I, Lagopoulos J et al (2007) Diffuse axonal injury in severe traumatic brain injury visualized using high-resolution diffusion tensor imaging. J Neurotrauma 24:753–765

Yoon S, Lee J, Kim S et al (2005) Evaluation of traumatic brain injured patients in correlation with functional status by localized 1H-MR spectroscopy. Clin Rehabil 19:209–215

Zakharova N (2013) Neuroimaging of structural and hemodynamic disturbances in severe traumatic brain injury (clinical CT – MRI studies). Dissertation, Burdenko neurosurgery institute, Moscow

Zakharova N, Potapov A, Pronin I et al (2006) Investigation of regional cerebral blood flow volume in patients with injuries and its consequences using CT-perfusion method. In: Abstracts of the European Society of Neuroradiology XXXI Congress, Geneva, 13 – 16 September 2006. Neuroradiology 48(Suppl 2):164

Zakharova N, Kornienko V, Potapov A, Pronin I et al (2007) Diffusion tensor MRI in severe diffuse axonal injury. In: Abstracts of the European Society of Neuroradiology XXXII Congress, Genoa, September 2007. Neuroradiology 49(Suppl 2):207

Zakharova N, Kornienko V, Potapov A et al (2008) Quantitative and qualitative evaluation of white matter damage by DT MRI and fibre tracking in diffuse axonal injury. In: Abstracts of the 13th EMN annual meeting, Heidelberg, 22–24 May 2008, p 48

Zakharova N, Potapov A, Kornienko V et al (2009) Diffusion tensor MRI of the white matter tracts in diffuse axonal injury. In: Abstracts of the 6th Black Sea Neurosurgical Congress, Istanbul, Sept 2009, p 178

Zakharova N, Potapov A, Kornienko V et al (2010a) Assessment of brain pathways in diffuse axonal injury using diffusion tensor MRI. Zh Vopr Neurokhir im NNBurdenko 2:3–9

Zakharova N, Potapov A, Kornienko V et al (2010b) Dynamic assessment of corpus callosum and corticospinal tracts structure using diffusion-tensor MRI in diffuse axonal injury. Zh Vopr Neurokhir im NNBurdenko 3:3–9

Clinical Evaluation and Neuroimaging Technologies

2

Contents

2.1 Clinical Material 25
2.2 Methods of Study 28
    2.2.1 Computed Tomography 28
    2.2.2 Magnetic Resonance Tomography 30
2.3 Statistical Analysis 33
References 33

2.1 Clinical Material

From 2003 to 2012, 4,235 patients with neurotrauma were admitted to Burdenko Neurosurgery Institute; 1,298 (31 %) patients were hospitalized in the acute period of trauma, while the remaining 2,937 (69 %) in subacute and chronic periods. Most patients (3,194; 75.4 %) had craniocerebral trauma.

The main indication for admission was severe neurotrauma which required high-technology methods of diagnosis, surgical interventions, neurological monitoring, and intensive care. Therefore, the overwhelming majority of patients (70 %) underwent neurosurgical interventions and the remaining patients (30 %) received conservative treatment.

This analysis included 208 patients (or 16 % of TBI patients) admitted to the institute in the acute period of trauma. They were examined in the acute, subacute, and delayed periods of brain trauma by generally accepted clinical and neuroimaging methods: CT, MRI (T1, T2, T2-FLAIR, gradient echo T2* imaging), also by advanced MRI sequences (DWI, DTI, 3D gradient echo – SWAN), as well as perfusion computed tomography (CT perfusion).

Patients' age varied from 6 to 72 years (mean age 28). Distributions of patients by age, mechanism, severity of injury, and outcome are listed in Tables 2.1, 2.2, and 2.3 and on Figs. 2.1, 2.2, and 2.3.

N. Zakharova et al., *Neuroimaging of Traumatic Brain Injury*,
DOI 10.1007/978-3-319-04355-5_2, © Springer International Publishing Switzerland 2014

Table 2.1 Characteristics of the examined groups of patients ($n=208$)

	Mean	Median	Minimum	Maximum	10th percentile	90th percentile	Standard deviation	Standard error
Age	30.65	28	6	72	17	49	13.12	0.91
GCS	8.04	7	3	15	4	13	3.396	0.24
GOS	3.51	3	1	5	2	5	1.077	0.07
Coma[a] duration, days	10.1	9	0	37	3	17	5.92	0.58

[a]Evaluated in comatose patients

Table 2.2 Distribution of patients based on the mechanism of damage

	1	2	3	4	5	6	
Mechanism	Falling from height	Assault	Motor vehicle	Motorcycle	Gunshot	Unknown	Total
n	25	35	118	18	5	7	208
Percentage	12	16.8	56.7	8.7	2.4	3.4	100

Table 2.3 Distribution of patients by Glasgow Outcome Scale

GOS	1	2	3	4	5	Total
n	12	16	77	61	42	208
Percentage	5.8	7.7	37	29.3	20.2	100

1, death; 2, vegetative state; 3, severe disability; 4, moderate disability; 5, good recovery

Fig. 2.1 Distribution of patients ($n=208$) by age

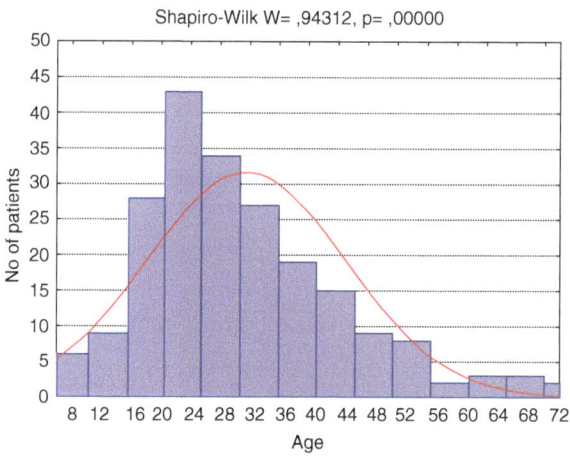

The main group (96.2 %) was presented by patients aged under 59, with half of them (54.8 %) being young people under 29 years old (Fig. 2.1); 62 of them were female (29.8 %) and 146 (70.2 %) male.

The main causes of head injury were traffic accidents (motor vehicle accidents: car or motorcycle) (65.4 %), assaults (16.8 %), and falls from one's own or great heights (12 %). The rest of the trauma mechanisms made up 5.8 % (Table 2.2).

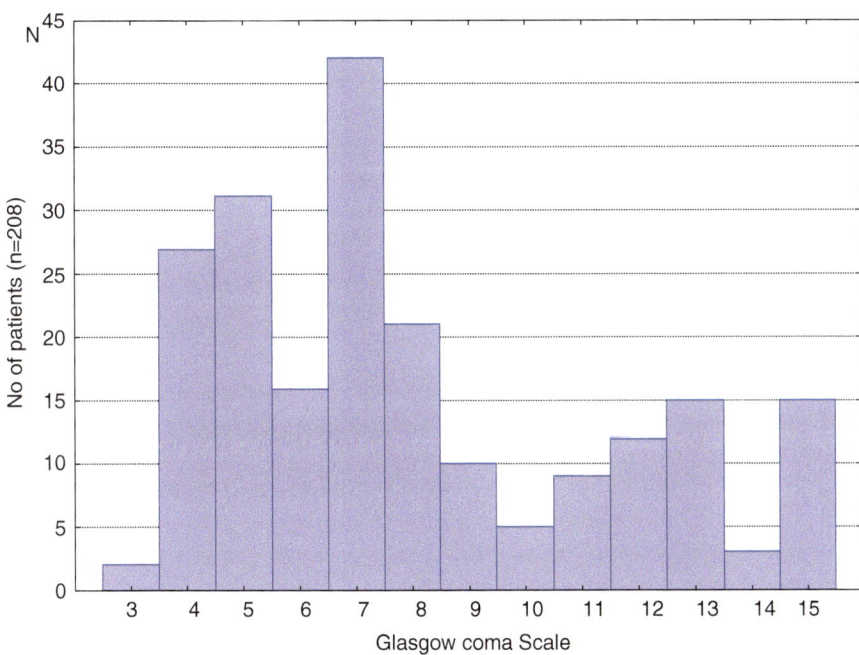

Fig. 2.2   Distribution of patients by Glasgow Coma Scale (GCS), $n = 208$

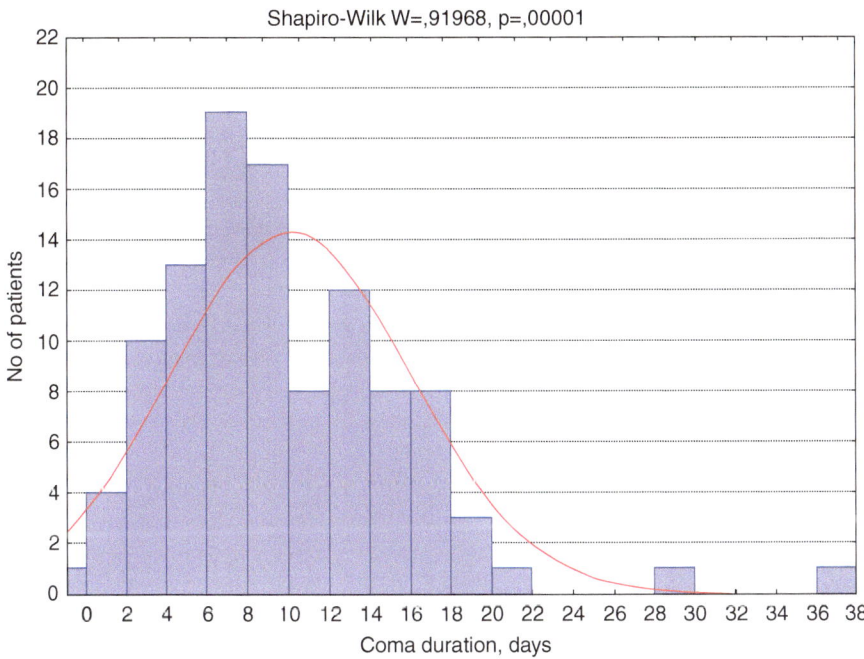

Fig. 2.3   Distribution of patients by coma duration ($n = 106$, number of patients with known duration). *Red curve* shows expected normal (Gaussian) distribution

Table 2.4 Distribution of patients based on the predominant type of injuries

Main types of injury	n	Percentage
Diffuse axonal injury (DAI)	45	21.6
Focal injury (contusions)	17	8.2
Diffuse + focal injury	33	15.9
Diffuse injury + intracranial hematoma (EDH/SDH/ICH)	23	11.1
Focal injury + intracranial hematoma (EDH/SDH/ICH)	37	17.8
Diffuse + focal injury + intracranial hematoma (EDH/SDH/ICH)	37	17.8
Gunshot injury of the head and brain	5	2.4
Other (concussion, CT-MRI norm)	11	5.2
Total	208	100

Patients' severity state at admission was evaluated by Glasgow Coma Scale (GCS) and varied from score 3 to 15 (average score, 7) (Teasdale and Jennett 1974). The majority of patients were in coma – GCS score ≤ 8 ($n = 139$; 66.8 %) (Fig. 2.2), with its duration widely varied (Fig. 2.3).

Evaluation of patients by Glasgow Outcome Scale (Jennett and Bond 1975) showed prevalence of severe disability, $n = 77$; 37 % (Table 2.3). However, there was no significant predominance of unfavorable outcome ($n = 105$; 50.5 %) over favorable one ($n = 103$; 49.5 %).

As is shown in Fig. 2.2, the distribution of patients by GCS on histogram differed from the normal one because the prevailing number of patients in the studied group had severe head trauma (GCS score ≤ 8). This explains the predominance of severe disability as outcome and makes it necessary to use such parameters as mean value, median, as well as 10th and 90th percentile in the statistical analysis.

Spearman's correlation showed an evidently significant correlation between outcome evaluated by GOS and severity of injury evaluated by GCS ($n = 208$, $R = 0.61$, $p < 0.01$) and suggests an adequate application of these two scales for evaluation of both severity of injury and its outcome.

Clinical and morphological diagnosis was based on the whole complex of data about mechanisms of injury, clinical state, neurological symptoms, CT and MRI findings, and dynamics of the clinical course (Table 2.4).

All patients were treated by TBI management protocol according to the evidence-based international guidelines (Bullock et al. 2000, 2006; Aarabi et al. 2001; Vos et al. 2002, 2012; Bratton et al. 2007). Neurological examination was reported to be useful in detecting motor or sensor deficits in patients without sedation.

2.2 Methods of Study

2.2.1 Computed Tomography

All patients underwent conventional computed tomography (CT) on admission and in dynamics. Assessment of regional cerebral blood flow (rCBF) by CT perfusion was performed in patients showing no allergy to iodinated contrast material (by relatives' words and informed consent) and after approval of CT protocols by the institute's ethical committee. As for CT perfusion it was a joint decision of neurosurgeons, neurologists, neurocritical care specialists, and neuroradiologists. It was suggested that measurements of rCBF were useful for choosing an optimal treatment tactics in each individual case. Guidelines for the safe use of CT perfusion were also considered (Wintermark et al. 2000; Wintermark 2010; Latchaw et al. 2002). Neither allergic reactions to the contrast material nor nephrotoxicity was marked in our series of patients.

Initially, each patient underwent a conventional unenhanced CT in order to determine a region of interest. The CT perfusion protocols included the following parameters for CT Brilliance-6 (Philips): scan type is continuous; 4-slices mode; total scanning time, 60 s; number of images, 60; scan rate, 1 image per second; number of slices × slice thickness, 4 × 6 mm; acquisition parameters, 90 kVp, 200 mA; and total number of images, 240; and for CT LightSpeed-16 (GE), scan type is cine mode; total scanning time, 50 s; number of images, 50; scan rate, 1 image per second; number of slices × image thickness, 4 × 5 mm; acquisition parameters, 80 kVp, 200 mA; and total number of images, 200.

The bolus of a 40.0 ml iodinated contrast material (370 mg/ml) was administered via the cubital or subclavian vein at a rate of 4 ml/s by using a power injector (and 20 ml of physiological saline after contrast agent) and 20 ml at 2 ml/s for children. The contrast was injected in 5 s before perfusion CT scanning for the cubital vein, and simultaneously with scanning for the subclavian vein. Perfusion CT data were post-processed at the workstation using a deconvolution algorithm. The arterial region of interest was manually selected in the anterior or middle cerebral arteries, while the venous one in the superior sagittal sinus (Kornienko and Pronin 2009).

CT perfusion effective radiation dose was 3.2 mSv, while the mean effective dose for the whole study (including localizer, conventional CT, CT perfusion) was 5.7 mSv.

There were qualitative assessments made for the three main perfusion parameters (mean ± 2 sd) extracted from maps: regional cerebral blood flow (rCBF in ml/100 g/min), regional cerebral blood volume (rCBV in ml/100 g), and mean transit time (MTT in seconds). In all cases, rCBF values were measured in three vascular regions in each hemisphere: anterior cerebral artery (ACA), middle cerebral artery (MCA), and posterior cerebral artery (PCA). ROI ranged from 300 to 1,200 mm^2. Besides, some additional rCBF assessments were performed in the damaged cortical-subcortical brain structures, symmetrical contralateral hemispheric structures, basal ganglia, thalami, and brain stem.

Four healthy volunteers without history of neurological disease or significant head trauma were studied using the same CT perfusion parameters, age ranged 21–36 (mean = 30) (Pronin et al. 2007).

In our study, as well as in Wintermark et al. (2004) study, ROIs included both gray and white matter, which have considerably different blood flow parameters. Thus, we used "normal" ranges for rCBF 28.6–69.0 (48.8 ± 10.1 ml/100 g/min), for rCBV 2.1–4.5 (3.3 ± 0.6 ml/100 g), and for MTT 2.7–5.9 (4.3 ± 0.8 s). Besides, peculiarities of rCBF in focal brain contusions and areas involving the main brain vascular structures were also considered.

According to the international guidelines for the management of severe TBI (Aarabi et al. 2001; Bullock et al. 2000, 2006; Potapov et al. 2003; Bratton et al. 2007), all comatose patients underwent invasive monitoring of the intracranial pressure (ICP) and direct recording of the arterial pressure (AP), which allowed a simultaneous monitoring of the cerebral perfusion pressure (CPP) (CPP=average AP – average ICP in mmHg). Presence and severity of intracranial hypertension were evaluated by the highest ICP values for the entire period of monitoring (2–12 days).

All patients with head injury underwent intensive therapy (including artificial lung ventilation) according to the international guidelines for the management of severe TBI (Bullock et al. 2000, 2006; Bratton et al. 2007).

Neurosurgical interventions on intracranial hematomas, impressed skull fractures, basal CSF leakage, as well as uni- or bilateral decompressive craniectomy (due to ICP increase and conservative treatment insufficiency) were performed according to the evidence-based guidelines for the surgical management of head injury. These procedures were described in the manuals, monographs, and other publications (Potapov and Gaytur 1998; Potapov et al. 2003, 2006; Aarabi et al. 2001; Bullock et al. 2006).

We used Marshall's classification (Marshall et al. 1991) for assessing the diffuse axonal injury (DAI) by CT scans.

Cortical-subcortical focal contusions were classified by CT grading into the following: (1), low density focus; (2), hemorrhagic zones of mixed density; and (3), intracerebral hematomas (Kornienko et al. 2003).

Presence and location of subarachnoid hemorrhages (SAHs) were described by the following signs: (0), absence; (1), convex; (2), basal; and (3), convex + basal. Intraventricular hemorrhage was also considered (presence or absence).

Deformations of mesencephalic cisterns were classified into the following types: (0), normal; (1), moderate narrowing; (2), asymmetric deformation; (3), severe narrowing and/or deformation; and (4), nonvisualized.

Outcome was evaluated by GOS (Glasgow Outcome Scale) in 3 and 6 months after injury: good recovery, moderate disability, severe disability, vegetative state, and death.

2.2.2 Magnetic Resonance Tomography

All studies were performed on 1.5T MRI (Signa Excite, GE) and 3T MRI (Signa HDxt GE) with the following MR sequences: T1, T2, T2-FLAIR, gradient echo images (2D T2* weighted, SWAN), and diffusion-weighted imaging (DWI) $b = 1,000$ s/mm^2 (all images were obtained in axial projection). For large-size intracerebral lesions or intracranial hematomas, we used sagittal and coronal images.

Diffusion-tensor MRI (DT MRI) in pulse sequence DW-SE-EPI (diffusion-weighted spin-echo single-shot echo-planar imaging) was taken in axial, sagittal, and coronal projections with the following parameters: for 1.5 T MRI, TR/TE; ms 8,000/93.2; 6 noncollinear directions of the diffusion gradient; NEX = 4; matrix, 256/256; slice thickness 5 mm, without gap; field of view = 240 mm, voxel size $1.9 \times 1.9 \times 5$ mm; 189 slices; and acquisition time, 4 min for 1 projection; and for 3 T MRI, TR/TE; ms, 8,000/96; 33 noncollinear directions of the diffusion gradient; NEX = 2; matrix, 256/256; slice thickness 4 mm, without gap; field of view =240 mm; voxel size $1.9 \times 1.9 \times 4$ mm; and acquisition time, 3 min 40 s for 1 projection.

Eighty-four MRI examinations were performed using DT-MRI (including repeated) for the analysis of the material presented in Chap. 4. Seventy-five examinations were performed on 1.5 T MRI (Signa Excite, GE) and 9 on 3 T MRI (Signa HDxt GE).

This study included eight healthy volunteers without history of neurological disorders and trauma, age range was 22–57 years (mean = 33; 5 males, 3 females).

Diffusion-tensor images were further transferred to the workstation equipped with specialized DTI and tractography processing software (FACT).

The apparent diffusion coefficient (ADC) and fractional anisotropy (FA) values were measured bilaterally: in the genu and splenium of the corpus callosum, in the posterior limb of the internal capsule (PLIC), cerebral peduncles, and at the level of the pons (along corticospinal tracts (CST). ROIs were drowned manually by a neuroradiologist in regions of interest, regardless of presence or absence of the damage foci. The number of included pixels corresponded to the respective dimension of the studied anatomical structures in any given slice. ADC and FA mean values with standard deviations were obtained for both patients with TBI and control group in the same anatomical structures.

Fractional anisotropy (FA) characterizes a spatial orientation of fibers and indicates how much higher the diffusivity is along some directions compared with others (Arfanakis et al. 2002). It is used as a quantitative indicator of diffusion anisotropy degree (Basser and Pierpaoli 1996; Pierpaoli et al. 1996; Sorensen et al. 1999). The FA values range from 0 to 1, where 0 is a maximal isotropic diffusion, as in a perfect sphere, and 1 the maximal anisotropic diffusion, as in a hypothetical case of a long cylinder of a minimal diameter (Huisman et al. 2004).

Diffusion anisotropy is distinct for each white matter structure. It reflects differences in fiber myelination, axonal density, and homogeneity in the axonal orientation (Mori et al. 2005). ADC (mean diffusivity) reflects the overall diffusion of water and is measured in mm^2/s (Fig. 2.4a).

Regions of high anisotropy (or with a high FA degree, e.g., the corpus callosum (CC)) are bright red on two-dimensional FA color maps. Regions of low anisotropy (or with a low FA degree, e.g., gray matter) are colored blue and yellow (Fig. 2.4b). The spatial direction of the mean anisotropic diffusion gradient in each voxel can be displayed by two-dimensional color-coding maps (Mori et al 2005). Red color indicates predominant right-left direction of the diffusion gradient (commissural fibers). Green indicates the predominant anterior-posterior direction (association fibers) and blue the superior-inferior direction (projection fibers) (Fig. 2.4c). 3D reconstructions of the corticospinal tracts and corpus callosum were performed in patients with TBI and healthy volunteers (Fig. 2.4d, e) (Huisman et al. 2004).

Three-dimensional diffusion tractography images of the CC fibers were obtained using the ROI positioned on the midsagittal plane around the CC on two-dimensional

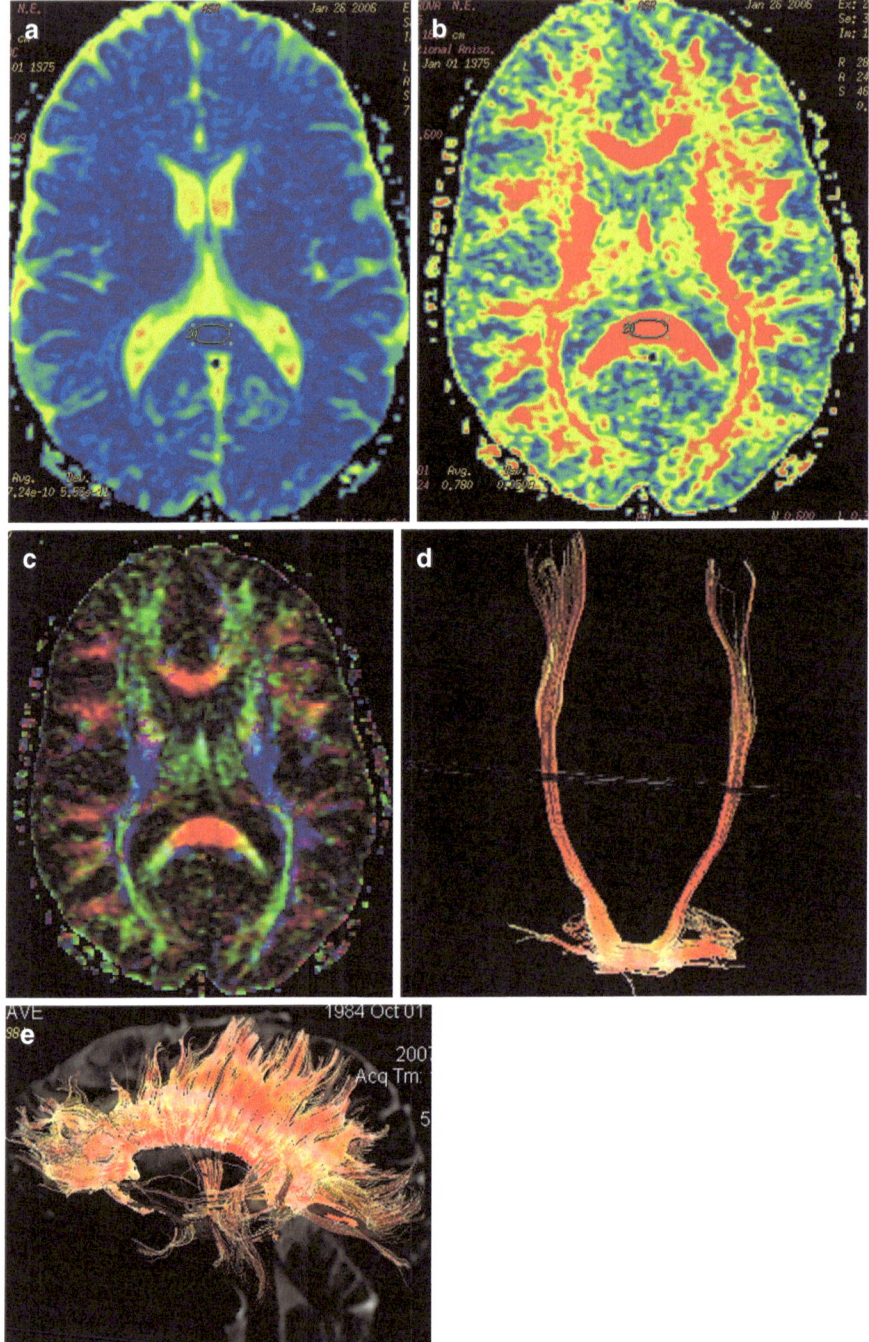

Fig. 2.4 Diffusion-tensor MRI in healthy volunteers: (**a**) apparent diffusion coefficient (ADC) map; (**b**) fractional anisotropy (FA) map; (**c**) color-coded orientation map; (**d**) 3D reconstruction of corticospinal tracts; (**e**) 3D reconstruction of the corpus callosum

FA maps. The seed ROIs for 3D images of corticospinal tracts (CSTs) were selected at the pons level at the regions of bilateral CST routes with their target positioned in the precentral gyrus of approximately 5–10 mm lower the motor cortex. Selection of commissural and projection tracts for 3D images depended on a comparatively easy detection of the CC on the midsagittal FA color maps, while CSTs have distinct unidirectionality.

2.3   Statistical Analysis

Statistical analysis was performed in MS Excel, Statistica, and R statistical packages for Windows. The calculations were made for absolute, relative, and rank values. All the statistical output parameters (minimum, maximum, mean values; standard errors; medians; standard deviations; 10th and 90th percentiles; Spearman's rank correlation coefficients; and p-values) were included in electronic tables. T-test was done to define statistically significant differences between measurements in right- and left-side areas of interest in patients and control subjects. The differences in groups by chi-square (χ^2) test of homogeneity and Wilcoxon tests were recognized as significant at the level of 0.05. Spearman's rank correlation coefficients were used to relate FA and ADC to clinical scales (GOS) and GCS to GOS.

References

Aarabi B, Alden T, Chesnut R et al (2001) Management and prognosis of penetrating brain injury. J Trauma 51:1–86

Arfanakis K, Haughton V, Carew J et al (2002) Diffusion tensor MR imaging in diffuse axonal injury. AJNR 23:794–802

Basser P, Pierpaoli C (1996) Microstructural and physiological features of tissues elucidated by quantitative – diffusion-tensor MRI. J Magn Reson 111:209–219

Bratton S, Bullock R, Chesnut R et al (2007) Guidelines for the management of severe traumatic brain injury. J Neurotrauma 24(7):55–58

Bullock R, Chesnut R, Clifton G et al (2000) Guidelines for management of severe traumatic brain injury. J Neurotrauma 17:451–553

Bullock R, Chesnut R, Ghajar J et al (2006) Guidelines for the surgical management of traumatic brain injury. Neurosurgery 58(Suppl 3):S2-1–S2-3

Huisman T, Schwamm L, Schaefer P et al (2004) Diffusion tensor imaging as potential biomarker of white matter injury in diffuse axonal injury. AJNR Am J Neuroradiol 25:370–376

Jennett B, Bond M (1975) Assessment of outcome after severe brain damage. Lancet 1:480–484

Kornienko V, Pronin I (eds) (2009) Diagnostic neuroradiology. Springer, Berlin/Heidelberg

Kornienko V, Potapov A, Pronin I, Zakharova N (2003) Diagnostic possibilities of computed and magnetic resonance imaging in traumatic brain injury. In: Potapov A, Likhterman L, Zelman V et al (eds) Evidence-based neurotraumatology. Andreeva TM, Moscow, pp 408–461

Latchaw R, Yones H, Hunter G et al (2002) Guidelines and recommendations for perfusion imaging in cerebral ischemia: a scientific statement for healthcare professionals by the writing group on perfusion imaging, from the Council on Cardiovascular Radiology of the American Heart Association. Stroke 34:1084–1104

Marshall L, Marshall S, Klauber M, Clark M (1991) A new classification of head injury based on computerized tomography. J Neurosurg 75:14–20

Mori S, Wakana S, Nagae-Poetscher L, van Zijl P (eds) (2005) MRI atlas of human white matter. Elsevier, Amsterdam

Pierpaoli C, Jezzard P, Basser P et al (1996) Diffusion tensor MR imaging of the human brain. Radiology 201:637–648

Potapov A, Gaytur E (1998) Biomechanics and basic links of pathogenesis of TBI. In: Konovalov A, Likhterman L, Potapov A (eds) Clinical guidelines on traumatic brain injury, vol 1. Antidor, Moscow, pp 152–165

Potapov A, Likhterman L, Zelman V, Kornienko V, Kravchuk A (eds) (2003) Evidence-based neurotraumatology. Andreeva TM, Moscow

Potapov A, Krylov V, Likhterman L et al (2006) Current guidelines for the diagnosis and treatment of severe brain injury. Zh Vopr Neurokhir im NNBurdenko 1:3–8

Pronin I, Fadeeva L, Zakharova N, Dolgushin M, Kornienko V (2007) Perfusion CT: evaluation of cerebral blood flow in normal subject. Med Visualiz 3:8–12

Sorensen A, Wu O, Copen W et al (1999) Human acute cerebral ischemia: detection of changes in water diffusion anisotropy by using MR imaging. Radiology 212:785–792

Teasdale G, Jennett B (1974) Assessment of coma and impaired consciousness. A practical scale. Lancet 2:81–85

Vos P, Battistin L, Birbamer G, Gerstenbrand F, Potapov A et al (2002) EFNS guideline on mild traumatic brain injury: report of an EFNS task force. Eur J Neurol 9(3):207–219

Vos P, Alexeenko Y, Battistin L, Ehler E, Gerstenbrand F, Muresanu D, Potapov A et al (2012) Mild traumatic brain injury. Eur J Neurol 19(2):191–198

Wintermark M (2010) FDA investigates the safety of brain perfusion CT. AJNR Am J Neuroradiol 31:2–3

Wintermark M, Maeder P, Verdun F et al (2000) Using 80kVp versus 120 Kvp in perfusion CT measurement of regional cerebral blood flow. AJNR Am J Neuroradiol 21:1881–1884

Wintermark M, van Melle G, Schnyder P et al (2004) Admission perfusion CT: prognostic value in patients with severe head trauma. Radiology 232:211–220

Contents

3.1 CT and MRI Data Comparison 35
3.2 MRI Classification of TBI 41
3.3 Discussion 61
References.. 66

3.1   CT and MRI Data Comparison

Comparison of CT and MRI data was performed in 43 patients with acute TBI (Table 3.1). The results of CT and MRI comparisons showed different sensitivity for detecting intracranial hemorrhages in the acute stage of TBI. MRI was evidently more sensitive than CT ($p<0.01$) in detecting deep brain structure damage, especially nonhemorrhagic, in subcortical white matter, corpus callosum, basal ganglia, thalami, and brain stem (Table 3.2).

Examples of CT and MRI sensitivity in acute and subacute phases of TBI are presented in Figs. 3.1, 3.2, 3.3, 3.4, 3.5, and 3.6.

As is shown in Fig. 3.1, T2-FLAIR MRI is accurate in visualizing corpus callosum damages, while T1 MRI and CT do not show these pathological changes.

Diffusion-weighted imaging (DWI) and diffusion-tensor imaging (DTI) are useful in visualizing water diffusion and anisotropy disturbances on ADC and FA maps. As is seen in Fig. 3.2, DWI shows change of intensity signal for the zones of restricted water diffusion and as such being indicative of local water electrolytic balance disturbances and cytotoxic edema development. Fractional anisotropy map and two-dimensional color-coded map demonstrate changes of anisotropy in the damage areas, while CT and T1 MRI do not reveal these damage zones.

This chapter has been contributed in collaboration with Eugenia Alexandrova and Gleb Danilov

N. Zakharova et al., *Neuroimaging of Traumatic Brain Injury*,
DOI 10.1007/978-3-319-04355-5_3, © Springer International Publishing Switzerland 2014

Table 3.1 Patient baseline characteristics (N = 43)

Gender: male/female	29/14
Patient's age, median value	29
GCS score, median value	7
GOS score, median value	3
Mechanism of trauma	
Traffic	31
Non-traffic	12

Table 3.2 Comparison of CT and MRI data in patients in the acute period of TBI

Injured structures and pathology	MRI data (Occurrence, percentage)	CT data (Occurrence, percentage)	p-value
Basal ganglia	40	14	0.003
Thalami	26	14	0.5
Corpus callosum	65	33	0.002
Brain stem	47	16	0.002
Focal contusions	77	70	0.5
ICH	23	23	0.7
SDH	56	33	0.02
EDH	5	12	0.23
SAH	88	88	0.9
IVH	35	26	0.3
Midline shift	33	37	0.7
Secondary ischemia	16	9	0.3

Dynamic DWI detects reversibility of posttraumatic cytotoxic edema by the end of third week after injury (Fig. 3.3). The data obtained show a 2–3-week time interval, when nonhemorrhagic parenchymatous changes caused by a cytotoxic edema can be revealed.

It is well known that CT is very sensitive for detection of acute hemorrhages, though in the ensuing period its diagnostic value decreases along with regression of hemorrhagic zone density. CT study in Fig. 3.4 was performed in 15 days after trauma and demonstrated only low-density contusions and midline shift, while MRI revealed hemorrhagic components of a focal contusion and subdural hematoma.

Our results have proved the generally accepted opinion that gradient echo, T2* GRE, 3D GRE, or SWAN (T2*-weighted angiography) are the most sensitive methods of neuroimaging of hemorrhages, especially microhemorrhages (Figs. 3.5 and 3.6). Its sensitivity was also rather high in the acute, subacute, and chronic periods of injury.

Case Report (Fig. 3.6)

M., 23 y.o., traffic accident. Diagnosis: severe combined trauma. Diffuse axonal injury: small hemorrhages in the white matter of hemispheres, basal ganglia, brain stem at the level of the medulla oblongata on the right, pons, midbrain from both sides. Subarachnoid hemorrhage, intraventricular hemorrhage. Skull vault fractures. Hemorrhage into the right frontal and supramaxillary sinuses. Heart contusion. Lung contusion.

On admission: GCS score 4. Length of coma, 37 days.

Four months after TBI: minimally conscious state (mutism with speech comprehension), severe mostly right-sided tetraparesis with hypertonus.

GOS: severe disability.

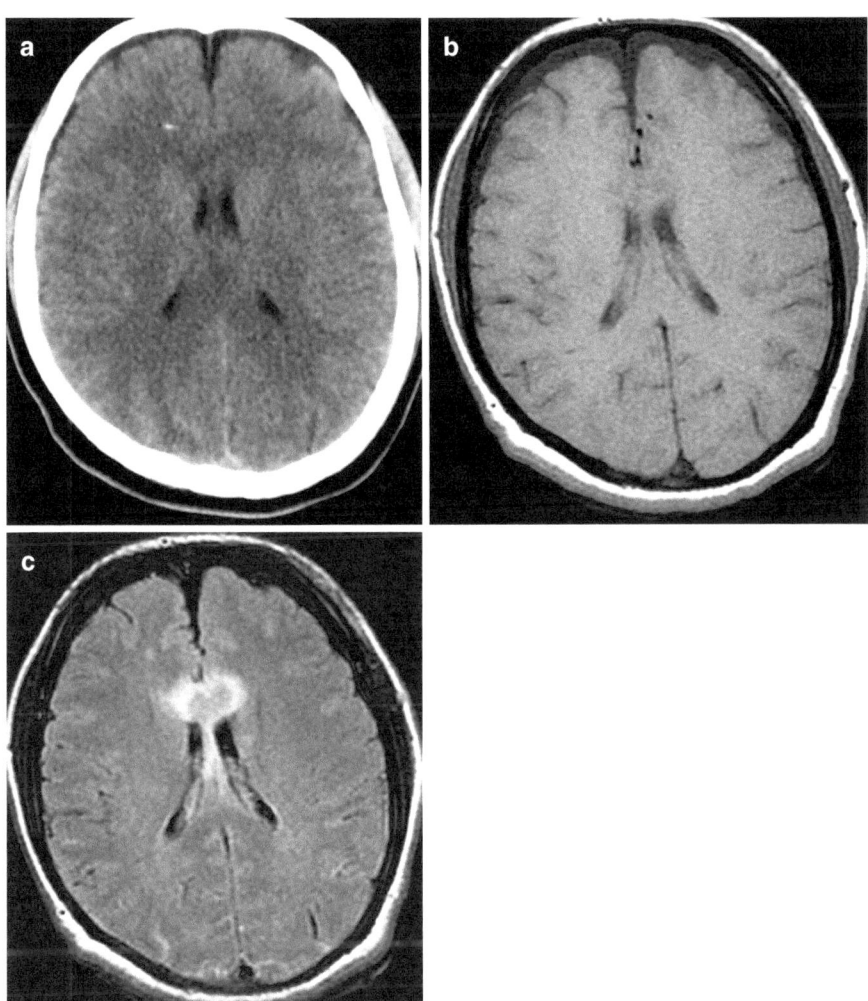

Fig. 3.1 CT and MRI data comparisons. Traffic accident. Five days after trauma. DAI: (**a**) CT – no visible changes, ICP sensor in the right frontal lobe; (**b**) T1WI – hygromas in frontal lobe regions; (**c**) T2-FLAIR clearly visualizes signs of corpus callosum damage

Thus, the data mentioned above show that MRI is more sensitive in detection of DAI with nonhemorrhagic lesions or microhemorrhages as well as intracranial hemorrhages and hematomas in subacute and chronic stages. That is why it seems reasonable to use not only CT but also advantages of different MRI sequences for a more detailed analysis of interrelation between TBI mechanisms, clinical status, and neuromorphological changes.

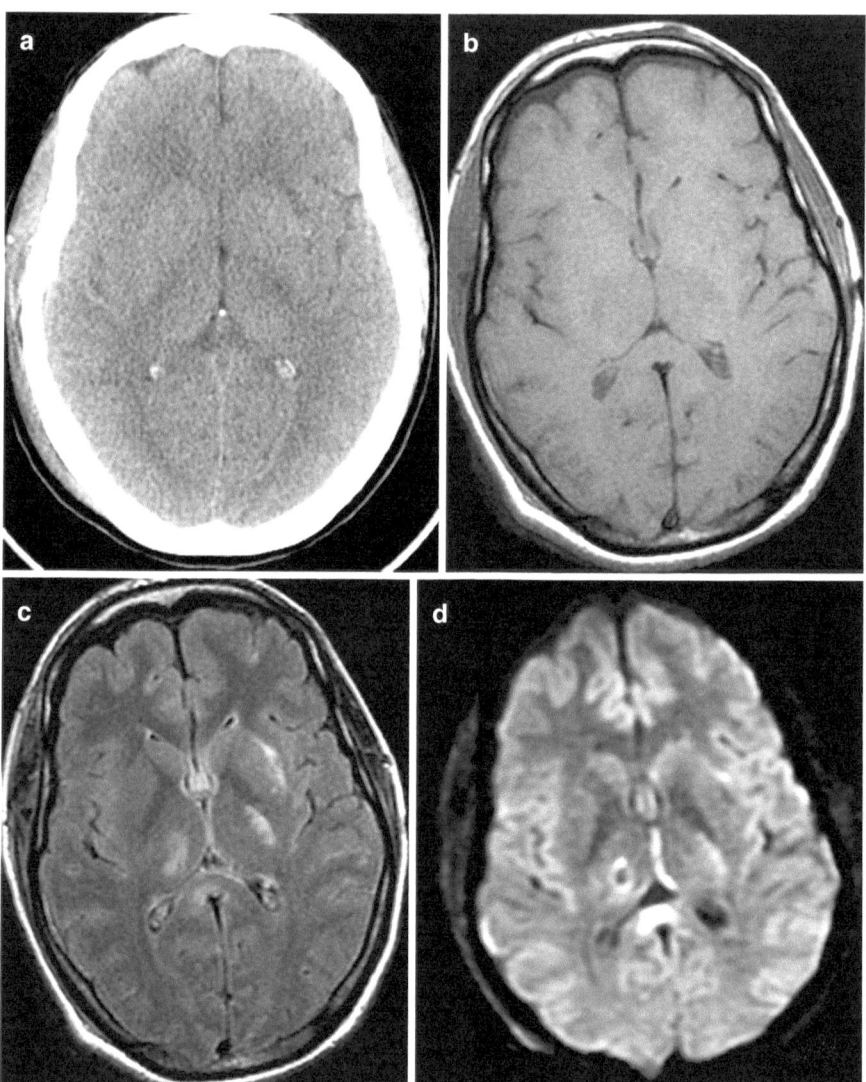

Fig. 3.2 Traffic accident. DAI. GCS – 5. CT and MRI data in 3 days after injury. CT (**a**) MRI (**b** T1WI; **c** T2-FLAIR; **d** diffusion-weighted imaging; **e** FA map, DT-MRI; **f** color-coded map, DT-MRI). Outcome: severe disability. See explanation in the text

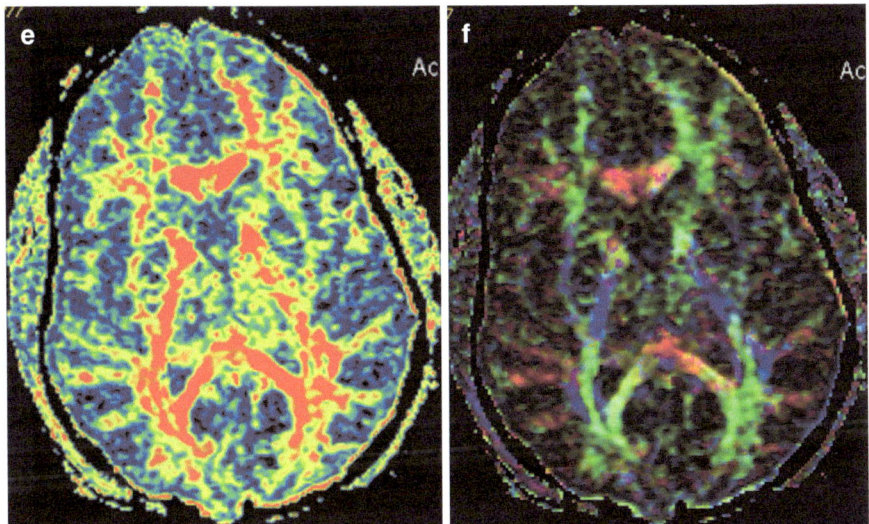

Fig. 3.2   (continued)

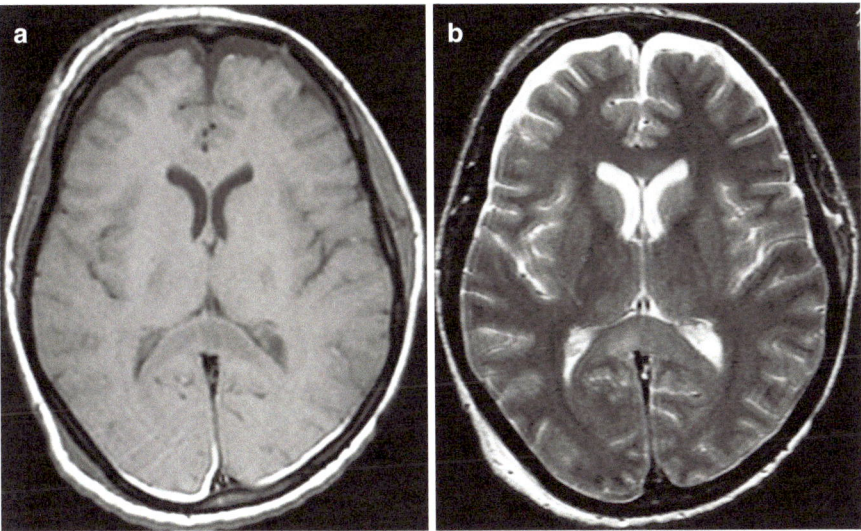

Fig. 3.3 Damage of the corpus callosum in DAI MRI (T1WI, T2WI, T2-FLAIR, DWI, ADC map) (**a–e**) in 8 days; (**f–i**) in 27 days after trauma. In 8 days, ADC values (**e**) in the splenium of the corpus callosum – $0.31 \pm 0.04 \times 10^{-3}$ mm²/s – indicate cytotoxic edema; in 27 days after trauma, (**i**) $0.684 \pm 0.09 \times 10^{-3}$ mm²/s (in norm, $0.7 \pm 0.075 \times 10^{-3}$ mm²/s)

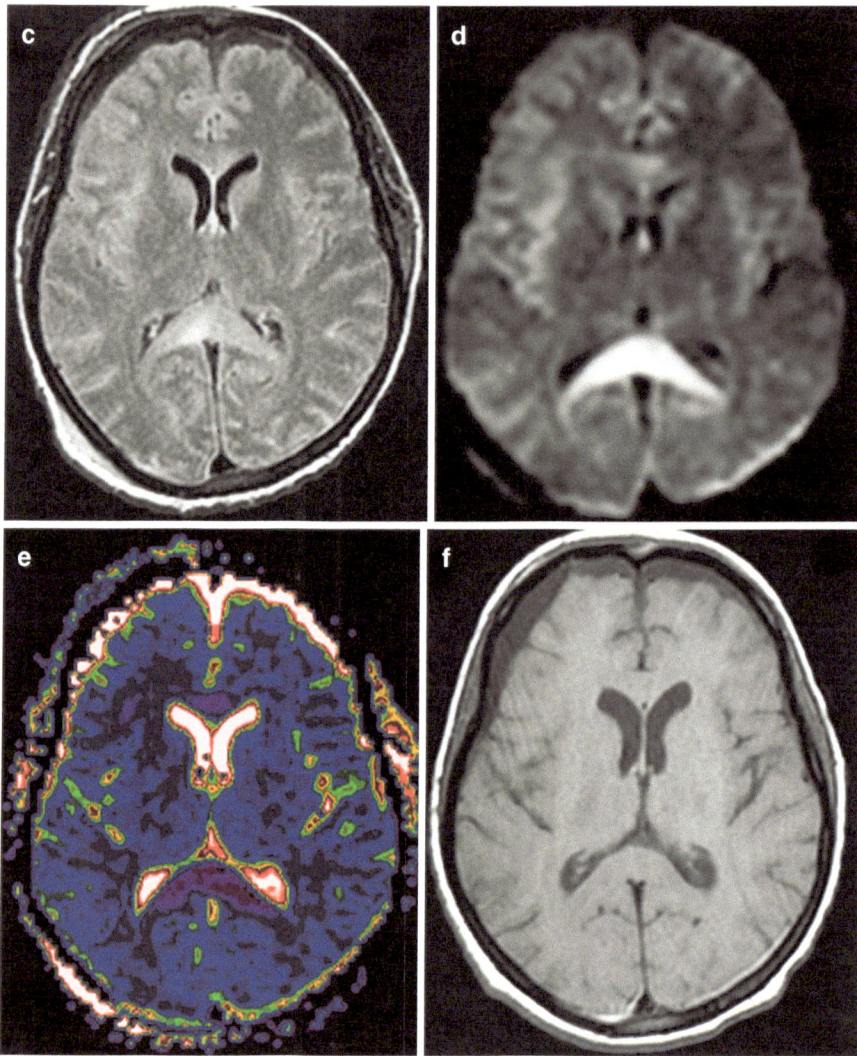

Fig. 3.3 (continued)

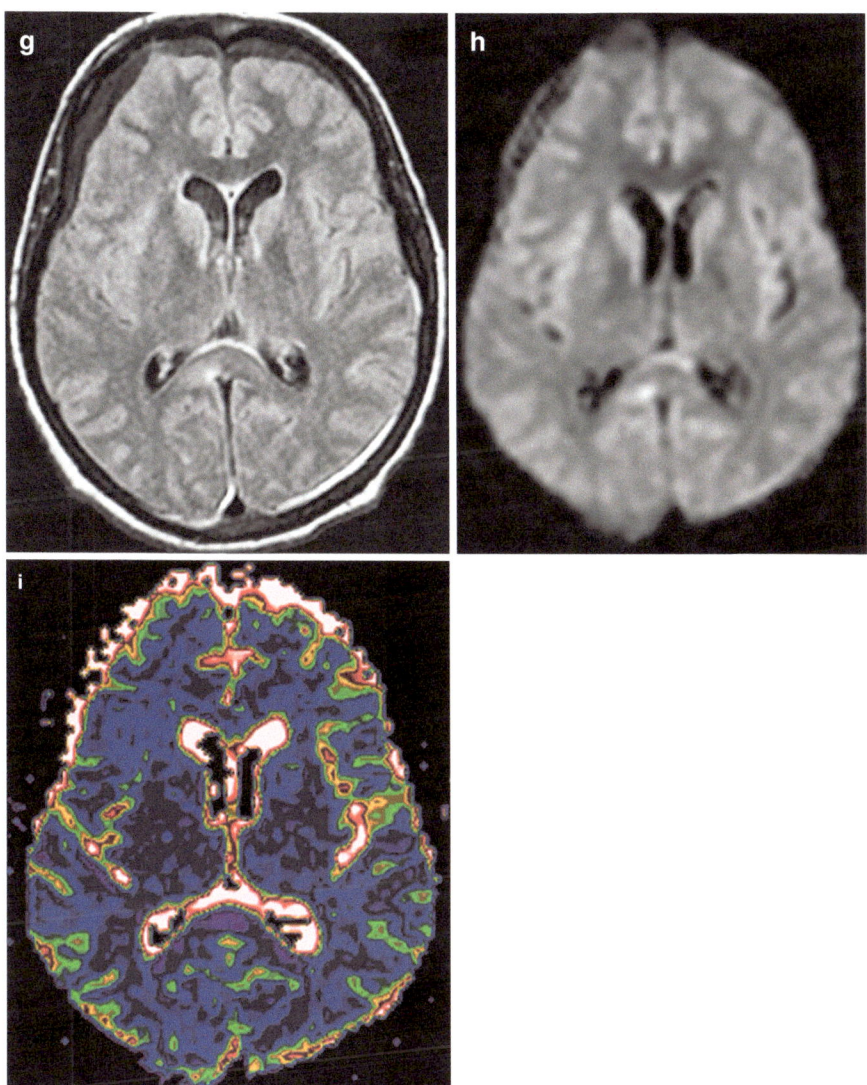

Fig. 3.3 (continued)

3.2   MRI Classification of TBI

The anatomy of the brain and its physiological, metabolic, neurotransmitter, and neurophysiological mechanisms responsible for structural and functional brain integrity, consciousness, and mental recovery are of a permanent interest for experimental and clinical neuroscientists (Castaigne et al. 1981; Munkle et al. 2000; Schiff and Plum 2000; McMillan and Herbert 2004; Lammi et al. 2005; Levin 2006;

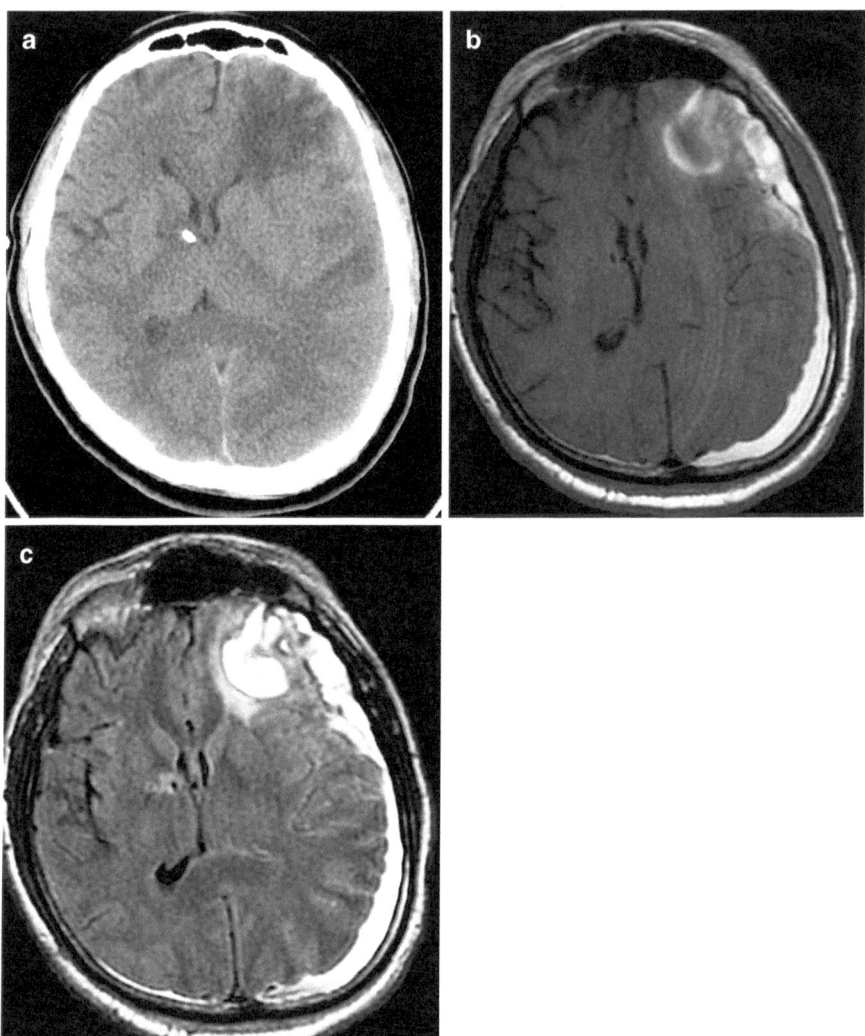

Fig. 3.4 CT (**a**) and MRI (**b** T1WI; **c** T2-FLAIR) data comparisons in cortical-subcortical focal contusion and subacute subdural hematoma (15 days after injury). See explanation in the text

Maxwell 2006; Owen et al. 2006; Posner et al. 2007; Augustenborg 2010; Alexandrova et al. 2011; Bragina et al. 2011; Oknina et al. 2011; Potapov and Likhterman 2011).

Development of modern neuroimaging technologies has opened up a new opportunity for studying this problem in normal and pathological conditions.

The first MRI classification of severe TBI was proposed by Firsching et al. (2001). They showed a high frequency of brain stem damage in patients with severe TBI in the acute phase. This classification was based on the location of brain stem

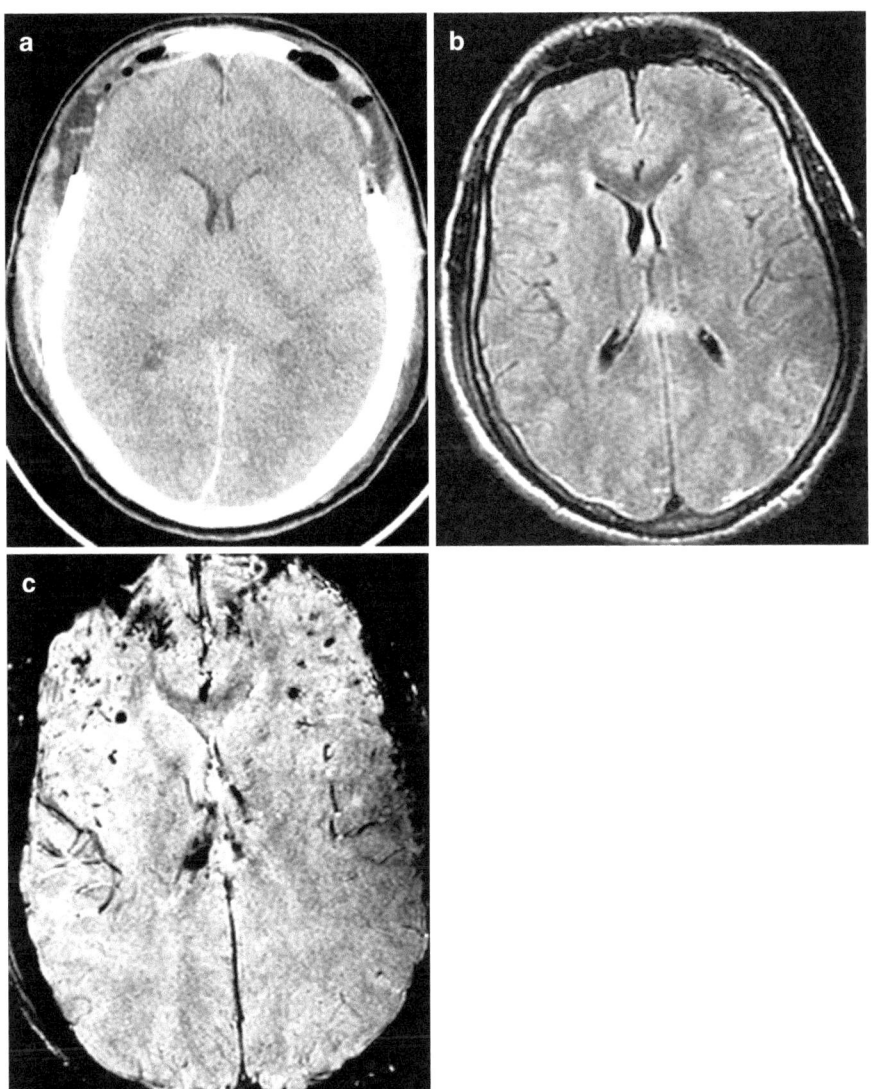

Fig. 3.5 Traffic accident. DAI. GCS, 8. CT (**a**) and MRI (**b** T2-FLAIR; **c** SWAN) data comparison in diffuse axonal injury with petechial hemorrhages and diffuse hemispheric edema. Increased intracranial hypertension, condition after decompressive bifrontal craniectomy. Outcome, moderate disability

injury using conventional MRI (T1, T2) sequences. The authors did not consider severity and location of supratentorial injuries and summarized all types of hemispheric damages in Grade I, regardless of deep subcortical structure involvement.

Mannion et al. (2007) analyzed 46 patients with severe TBI using T2, FLAIR, and T2*GRE MRI sequences. Unfavorable outcome was observed in 55 % of

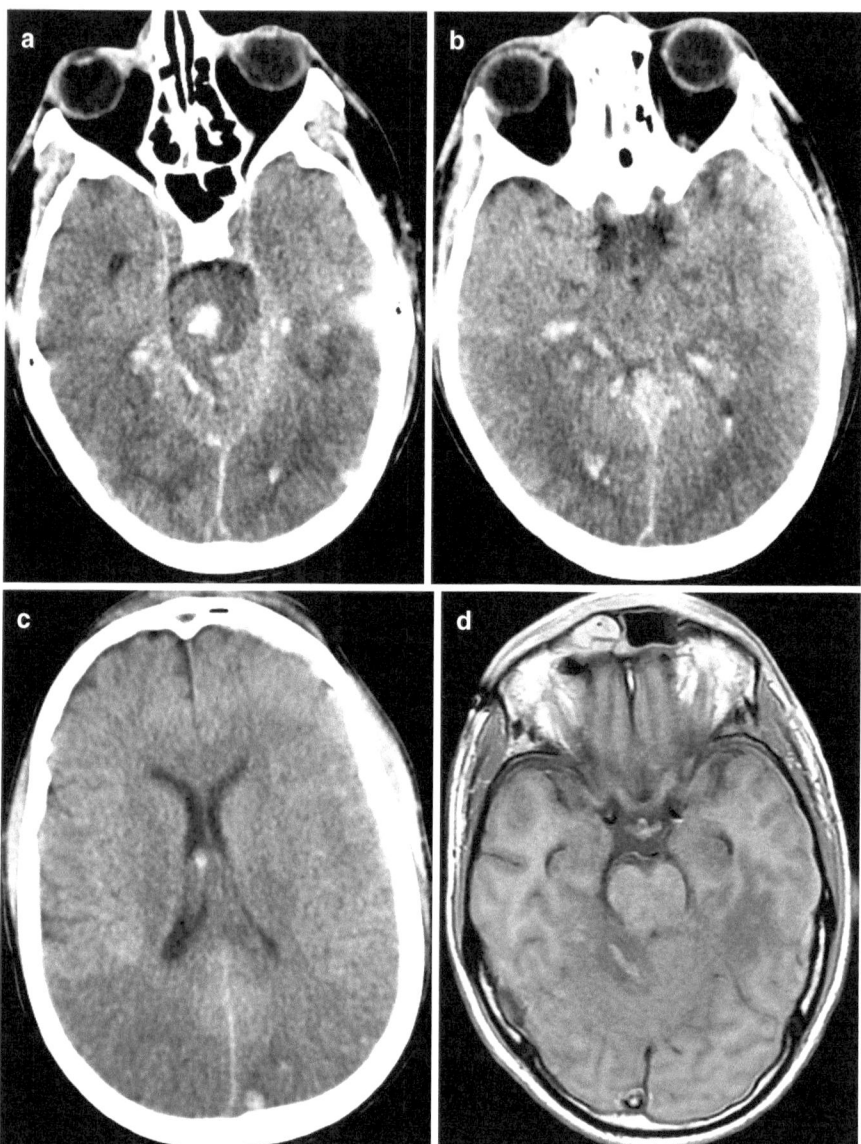

Fig. 3.6 Traffic accident. DAI. GCS, 4. CT and MRI studies in the first day after injury. Coma duration, 37 days. Outcome, severe disability. CT (**a–c**) and MRI (T1WI, **d, e**; T2WI, **f, g**) data comparison; SWAN modality (**h, i**) shows higher sensitivity in petechial hemorrhage detection

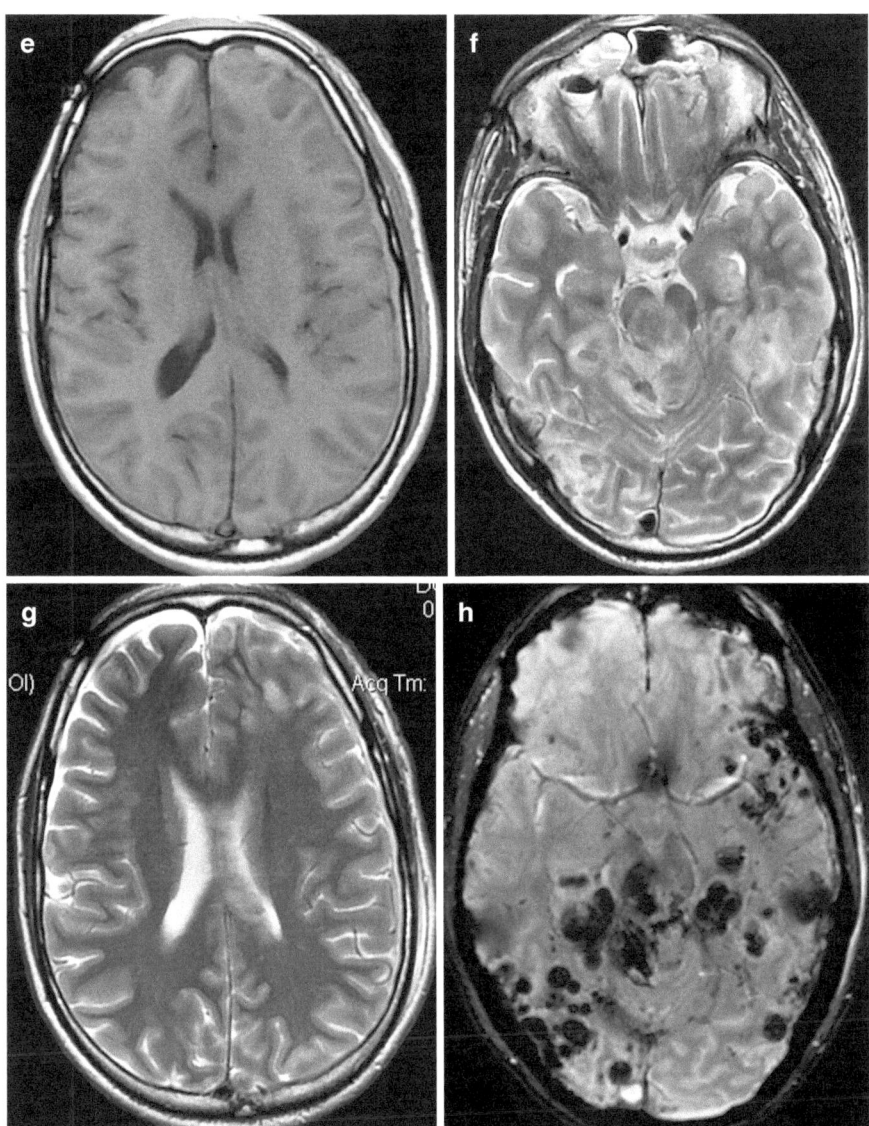

Fig. 3.6 (continued)

Fig. 3.6 (continued)

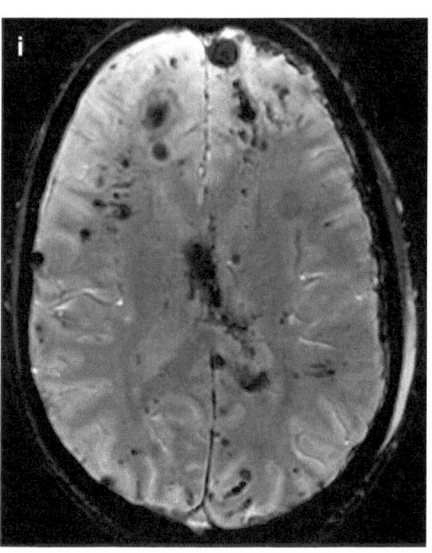

patients with supratentorial damages only and in 85 % (11 of 13 patients) of patients with brain stem damages. Though the correlation between brain stem lesions and outcome was significant, the authors did not regard brain stem damage as an absolute prognostic factor of unfavorable outcome.

These and other publications reported mostly severe TBI cases based on a limited spectrum of MRI sequences. At the same time, neither qualitative analysis of coma nor comparisons of brain stem injury rates in mild and moderate TBI have been given.

Today it is still unclear what localizations and severity of traumatic brain injury may cause disorders of consciousness and development of coma with a variable depth and duration. It equally applies not only to the brain stem but also to the thalamus, basal ganglia, corpus callosum, and cortical-subcortical structures.

To answer this question 162 patients with acute and subacute TBI of various severity were examined by different sequences of MRI (T1, T2, T2-FLAIR, DWI, T2* gradient echo, SWAN). Patients' age varied 8–72 (mean age 29.6 ± 12.8 years). The main group of patients aged 15–59 years (91.35 %); half of the injured were young people aged 8–26 years (Fig. 3.7); 71 patients (48 %) underwent MRI within 1–7 days after injury, 33 % within 8–14 days, and 19 % within 15–21 days after injury (average 8.7 ± 5.7 days).

MRI data were used for a more differentiated evaluation of hemispheric and brain stem damages. This analysis permitted us to propose MRI grades. The number of patients classified by this extended MRI gradation is depicted in Table 3.3; each next grade may include the lesions of previous grades.

The histogram (Fig. 3.8) shows distribution of patients by Glasgow Coma Scale (GCS) with its score varied from 3 to 15 (average 8 ± 3; median 7; 10 and 90

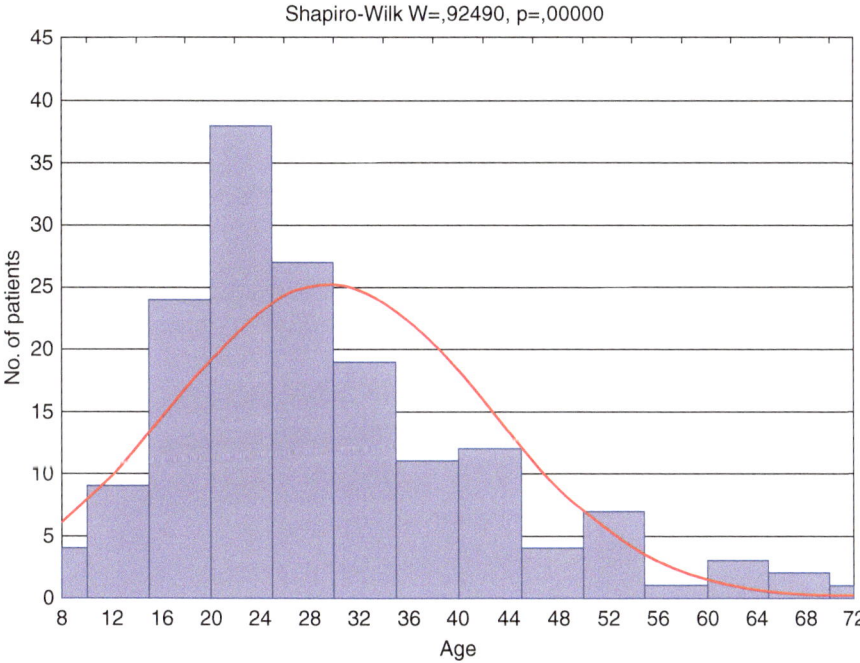

Fig. 3.7 Distribution of patients by age ($n = 162$). *Red curve* shows expected normal (Gaussian) distribution

Descriptive statistics

	N	Mean	Median	Minimum	Maximum	10th percentile	90th percentile	Std. dev.	Standard error
Age	162	29.61	26	8	72	16	48	12.79	1.005

Table 3.3 Number of patients evaluated by extended MRI gradation ($n = 162$)

Injury level	Occurrence (n, %)
1. No signs of parenchymatous lesions	10 (6.2)
2. Cortical-subcortical lesions	31 (19.1)
3. Corpus callosum damage ± 2	24 (14.8)
4. Uni- or bilateral damage of the basal ganglia and/or thalami ± (2–3)	21 (13)
5. Unilateral brain stem damage at different levels ± (2–4)	29 (17.9)
6. Bilateral midbrain damage ± (2–4)	30 (18.5)
7. Bilateral pons damage ± (2–6)	15 (9.3)
8. Bilateral medulla oblongata damage + (2–7)	2 (1.2)

percentile, scores 4 and 13 correspondingly); 65 % of 162 patients were in coma (GCS ≤ 8), 18 % had GCS score 9–12, and 17 % GCS score 13–15.

The histograms (Figs. 3.8 and 3.9) show patient distribution by GCS and GOS different from the normal due to severe TBI predominance in the analyzed groups of patients (GCS ≤ 8), and hence, severe disability prevailed in groups of outcome.

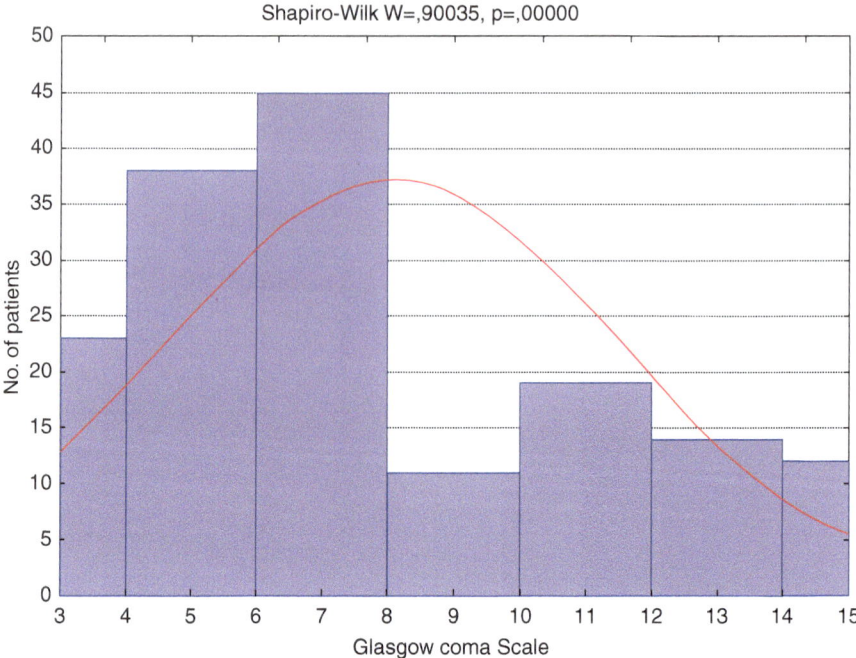

Fig. 3.8 Distribution of patients by Glasgow Coma Scale (GCS), $n=162$. *Red curve* shows expected normal (Gaussian) distribution

Descriptive statistics

	N	Mean	Median	Minimum	Maximum	10th percentile	90th percentile	Std. dev.	Standard error
GCS	162	8.07	7	3	15	4	13	3.4697	0.273

As seen from Table 3.4 the majority (65 %) of the analyzed patients was in coma; coma rate depended on levels and localization of hemispheric deep structures and brain stem lesions.

Spearman's rank correlation analysis revealed a statistically significant correlation between outcome evaluated by GOS and severity evaluated by GCS in a group of patients with MRI performed within 1–21 days after trauma ($R=0.63$, $p<0.001$). It allowed using these important clinical and prognostic indicators (Glasgow Coma Scale and Glasgow Outcome Scale) for further analysis of trauma mechanisms, CT and MRI data, etc.

An evident correlation ($R=-0.44$, $p<0.01$) between GCS and length of coma was revealed in comatose patients with severe TBI (GCS ≤ 8) and a low correlation ($R=-0.22$, $p<0.04$) between GCS and CT categories of severe diffuse injury proposed by Marshall et al. (1991).

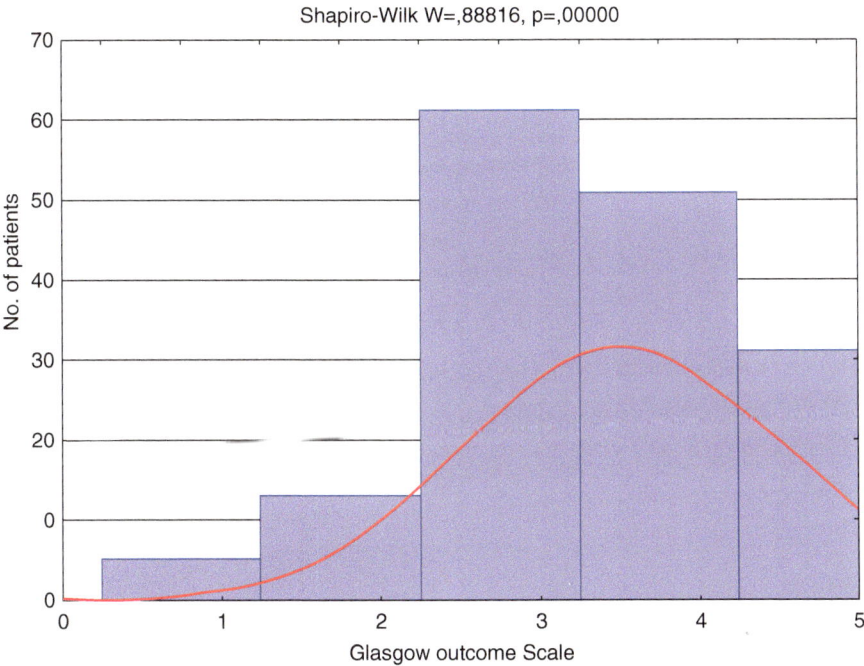

Fig. 3.9 Distribution of patients by Glasgow Outcome Scale (GOS), $n = 162$. *Red curve* shows expected normal (Gaussian) distribution

Descriptive statistics

	N	Mean	Median	Minimum	Maximum	10th percentile	90th percentile	Std. dev.	Standard error
GOS	162	3.55	4	1	5	2	5	0.9927	0.078

Table 3.4 Occurrence of patients in coma (GCS ≤ 8) and unfavorable outcome (GCS 1–3) in analyzed groups of patients, divided by extended MRI gradation

	Total	GCS ≤ 8		GOS 1–3	
Injury level	n	n	%	n	%
1. No signs of parenchymatous lesions	10	1	10	0	0
2. Cortical-subcortical lesions	31	9	29	4	13
3. Corpus callosum damage ± 2	24	16	67	7	29
4. Uni- or bilateral damage of the basal ganglia and/or thalami ± (2–3)	21	12	57	10	48
5. Unilateral brain stem damage at different levels ± (2–4)	29	25	86	15	52
6. Bilateral midbrain damage ± (2–4)	30	28	93	27	90
7. Bilateral pons damage ± (2–6)	15	14	93	15	100
8. Bilateral medulla oblongata damage ± (2–7)	2	1	50	1	50
Total	162	106	65	79	49

Table 3.5 Clinical characteristics of patients with different causes of trauma ($n = 162$)

	1	2	3	4	5	
Clinical characteristics	Falls	Assault	Motor vehicle	Motorcycle	Others	p-values in groups
n	14	27	102	14	5	
Age (mean)	36	33	28	28	27	(2 and 3) $p = 0.03$
GCS (mean)	11	11	7	7	9	(1 and 3) $p < 0.04$
						(2 and 3) $p < 0.0001$
GOS (mean)	4	4	3	3	4	(1 and 2) $p < 0.01$
						(1 and 3) $p < 0.01$
						(1 and 4) $p < 0.01$
						(3 and 4) $p < 0.001$
Firsching's grades	1	1	2	2	1	(1 and 3) $p < 0.01$
(mean, n)	$n = 13$	$n = 26$	$n = 101$	$n = 14$	$n = 5$	(2 and 3) $p < 0.000$
						(3 and 4) $p < 0.0001$
Extended MRI grading	3	3	5	5	3	(1 and 3) $p < 0.001$
(mean, n)	$n = 13$	$n = 26$	$n = 101$	$n = 14$	$n = 5$	(2 and 3) $p < 0.0001$

Significant correlations between MRI four-grade classification proposed by Firsching et al. (2001), GCS ($R = -0.59$, $p < 0.001$), and GOS ($R = -0.68$, $p < 0.001$) were revealed in the whole group of patients ($n = 162$) with different TBI severity.

The most frequent causes of TBI were traffic accidents (motorcycle, motor vehicle, etc.) (71.6 %), followed by assaults (16.6 %) and falls from one's own or great heights (8.6 %); other cases made up 3 % (Table 3.5). According to GCS evaluations, motor vehicle and motorcycle crashes lead to a more severe injury and less favorable outcome ($p < 0.01$) compared to other causes of trauma (Table 3.5), what may be explained by the dominating acceleration-deceleration mechanisms.

MRI data analysis showed that the most frequent cause of damage to deep brain structures (basal ganglia, thalamus, corpus callosum, and brain stem) was car accidents ($p < 0.05$), compared to other causes of trauma (Table 3.6). Injury of deep brain structures is known to be typical for DAI. Our results have confirmed that the leading cause of this type of injury is motor vehicle accidents.

Corpus callosum (CC) injury rate was slightly higher for age groups under 44. All age groups showed high rate of subarachnoid hemorrhages (Table 3.7).

Table 3.8 demonstrates significantly higher rate of brain stem injury (grades 4–8) for traffic accidents ($p < 0.01$) than for other trauma mechanisms.

Our data revealed a higher correlation between eight-grade MRI classification, GCS, and GOS ($R = -0.62$, $p < 0.01$ and $R = -0.72$, $p < 0.01$, correspondingly) compared to a four-grade classification by Firsching et al. (2001). This correlation is demonstrated on three-dimensional histograms (Figs. 3.10 and 3.11) and in Table 3.9. The data obtained have shown a high prognostic value of the new MRI classification of TBI levels and localizations.

Table 3.6 Injured brain structures (MRI data) in patients with different causes of TBI (data are numbers of patients, $n = 162$)

	1	2	3	4	5	
MRI data (injured structures and pathology)	Falls	Assault	Motor vehicle	Motorcycle	Others	p-values in groups
Basal ganglia	2	3	50	7	0	(2 and 4) $p < 0.01$ (2 and 3) $p < 0.001$
Thalami	1	1	39	6	1	(2 and 3) $p < 0.01$ (2 and 4) $p < 0.01$
Corpus callosum	3	8	87	11	2	(1 and 3) $p < 0.0001$ (1 and 4) $p < 0.01$ (2 and 3) $p < 0.0001$ (2 and 4) $p < 0.01$
Brain stem	3	5	59	8	2	(1 and 3) $p < 0.001$ (3 and 5) $p < 0.0001$ (2 and 4) $p < 0.05$
ICH	2	2	17	1	0	No significant difference
SDH	9	15	29	10	2	(1 and 3) $p < 0.05$ (2 and 3) $p < 0.05$ (3 and 4) $p < 0.05$
EDH	1	4	9	1	1	No significant difference
SAH	12	18	76	11	4	No significant difference
IVH	1	3	31	3	2	No significant difference
Midline shift	5	12	21	5	2	(3 and 4) $p < 0.05$
Basal cistern compression	5	13	70	12	3	(1 and 4) $p < 0.05$ (3 and 4) $p < 0.05$
Total	14	27	102	14	5	

Table 3.7 MRI data in different age groups, percentage ($n = 162$)

Age group	0–14	15–29	30–44	45–59	60–72
n (%)	8 (4.9)	88 (54.3)	46 (28.4)	14 (8.6)	6 (3.7)
MRI data					
Basal ganglia	50	51.1	34.8	21.4	50
Thalami	37.5	47.7	19.5	14.3	16.7
Corpus callosum	75	82.9	69.5	42.8	50
Brain stem	87.5	50	47.8	84.6	100
ICH	12.5	10.2	15.2	28.6	16.7
SDH	25	37.5	43.5	57.1	33.3
EDH	25	10.2	10.9	0	0
SAH	75	89.8	46.6	92.9	100
IVH	37.5	25	17.4	35.7	33.3
Basal cistern compression	62.5	69.3	43.5	42.9	50
Secondary ischemia	0	18.4	6.5	14.3	0

Table 3.8 Causes of trauma for each group of patients divided by extended MRI grading (2 patients with grade 8 were included into grade 7)

	1	2	3	4	5
Injury level	Falls	Assault	Motor vehicle	Motorcycle	Others
1	2	3	4	0	1
2	6	14	8	2	1
3	2	3	17	0	1
4	1	2	14	3	0
5	1	4	18	5	1
6	0	0	27	2	1
7/8	2	1	14	1	0
Total	14 (8.6 %)	27 (16.7 %)	102(63 %)	14 (8.6 %)	5 (3.1 %)

Table 3.9 Correlation between age, mechanism of trauma, GCS, GOS, Firsching's classification, and extended MRI grading

	Age	Mechanism of trauma	GCS	GOS
Age	1.000	−0.186*	0.150	−0.082
Mechanism of trauma	−0.186*	1.000	−0.352*	−0.192*
GCS	0.150	−0.352*	1.000	0.638*
GOS	−0.083	−0.192*	0.638*	1.000
Firsching's classification	−0.023	0.239*	−0.589*	−0.678*
Extended MRI grading	−0.065	0.309*	−0.624*	−0.717*

*Statistically significant correlation, $p < 0.05$

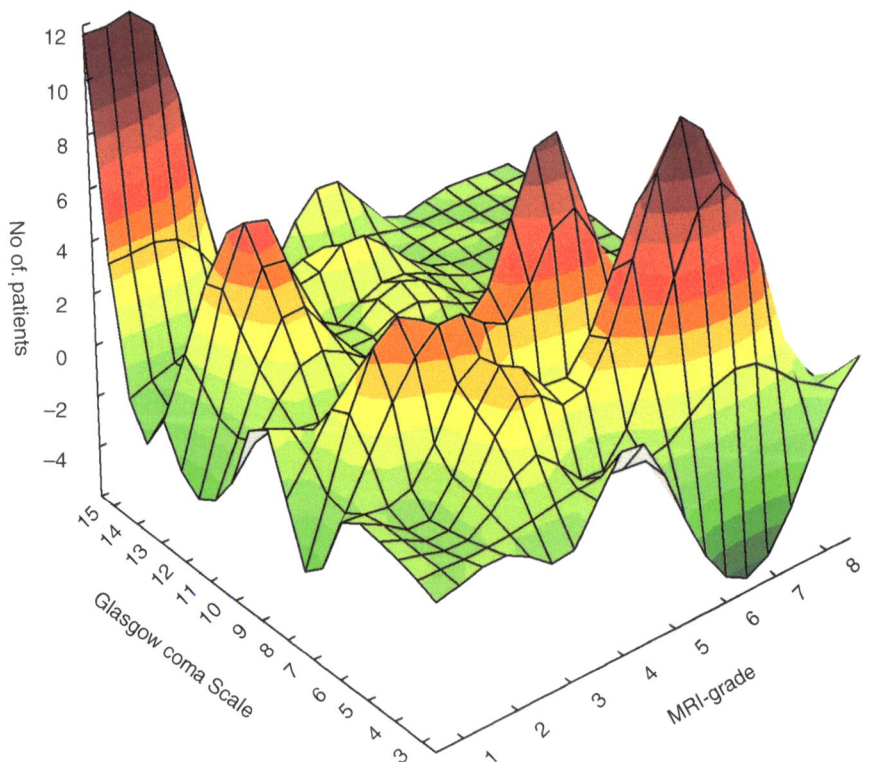

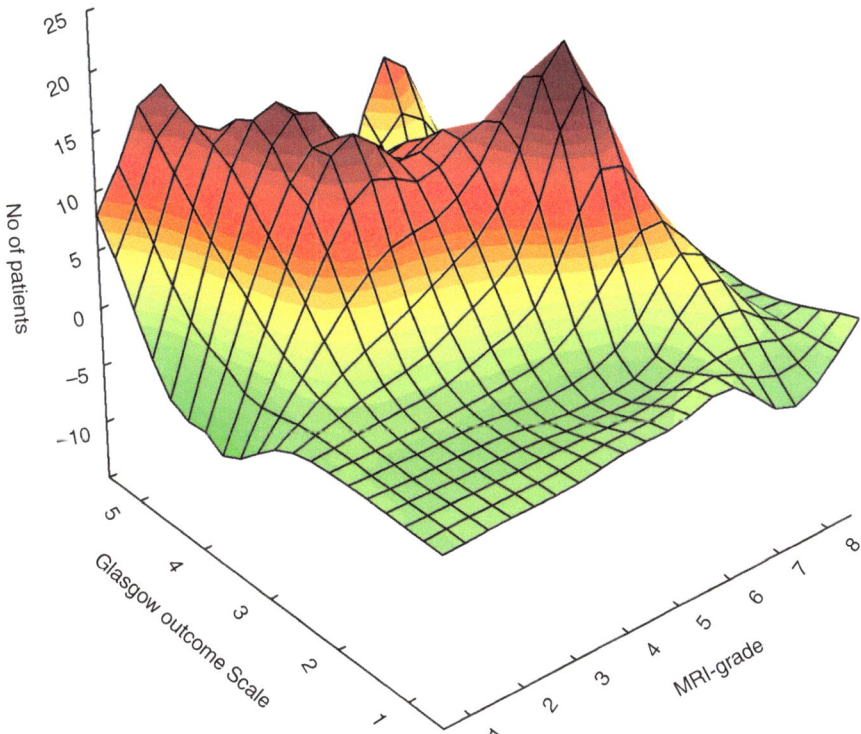

Fig. 3.11 Bivariant histogram of patient distribution ($n=162$) by Glasgow Outcome Scale and new eight-grade scale of injury localization and level

The scores by proposed MRI grading scale better correlate with GCS and GOS than the four-grade scale esteems do (Table 3.9). This is clearly seen in proportions of patients in comatose state and with subsequent unfavorable outcome depending on the traumatic damage location demonstrated on the graph (Fig. 3.12). The relationship between the brain stem and thalamus injury rates and GCS severity is represented on Fig. 3.13.

The MRI cases presented below are useful for evaluating levels and locations of injuries in patients with acute TBI (Figs. 3.14, 3.15, 3.16, 3.17, and 3.18).

As an example of primary bilateral injury of the medulla oblongata, we report the case of a 22-year-old female who sustained TBI in a car accident. She was obnubilated (GCS score 11) on admission to hospital and had severe brain stem damage symptoms, episodes of apnea requiring intubation and prolonged artificial ventilation, and tetraparesis. The patient was transferred to Burdenko Institute. MRI revealed damages of the basal ganglia, midbrain, pons, and medulla oblongata

Fig. 3.10 Bivariant histogram of patient distribution ($n=162$) by Glasgow Coma Scale and new eight-grade scale of injury localization and level

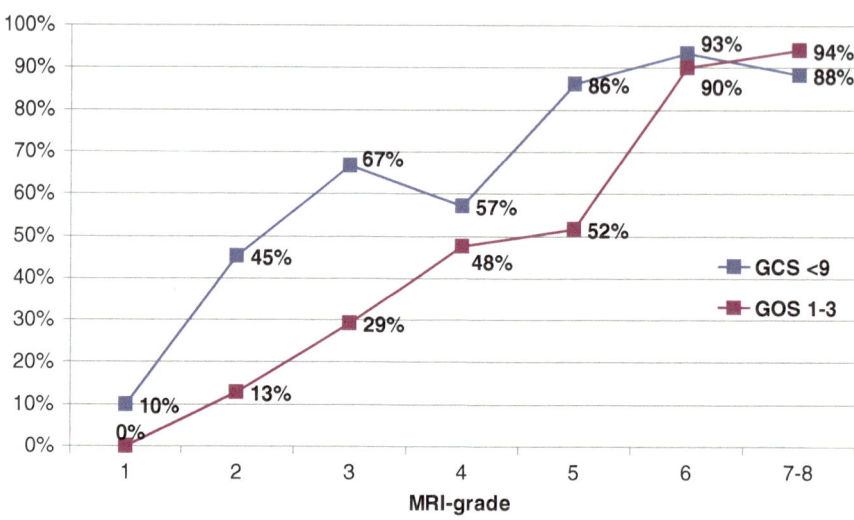

Fig. 3.12   The rate of comatose state and unfavorable outcomes in patients with different levels of brain damage (by MRI data). Two patients with bilateral damage of the medulla oblongata (grade 8) are combined with patients of grade 7 (bilateral pons damage)

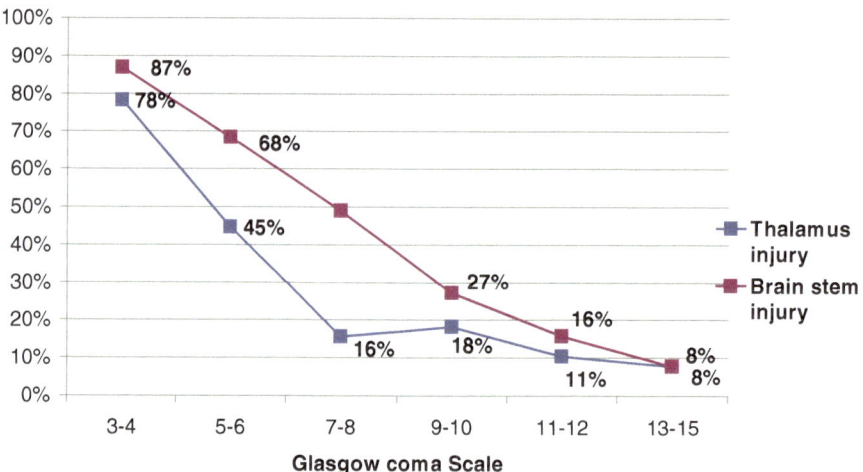

Fig. 3.13   Brain stem and thalamus injury rates (by MRI data) in brain trauma of different severity (by GCS)

(Fig. 3.19). Intensive care with artificial ventilation support resulted in restored adequate spontaneous respiration, brain stem symptoms, and tetraparesis regression. She had clear consciousness state, mild brain stem symptoms, and tetrasyndrome (mild bilateral pyramidal insufficiency) at discharge.

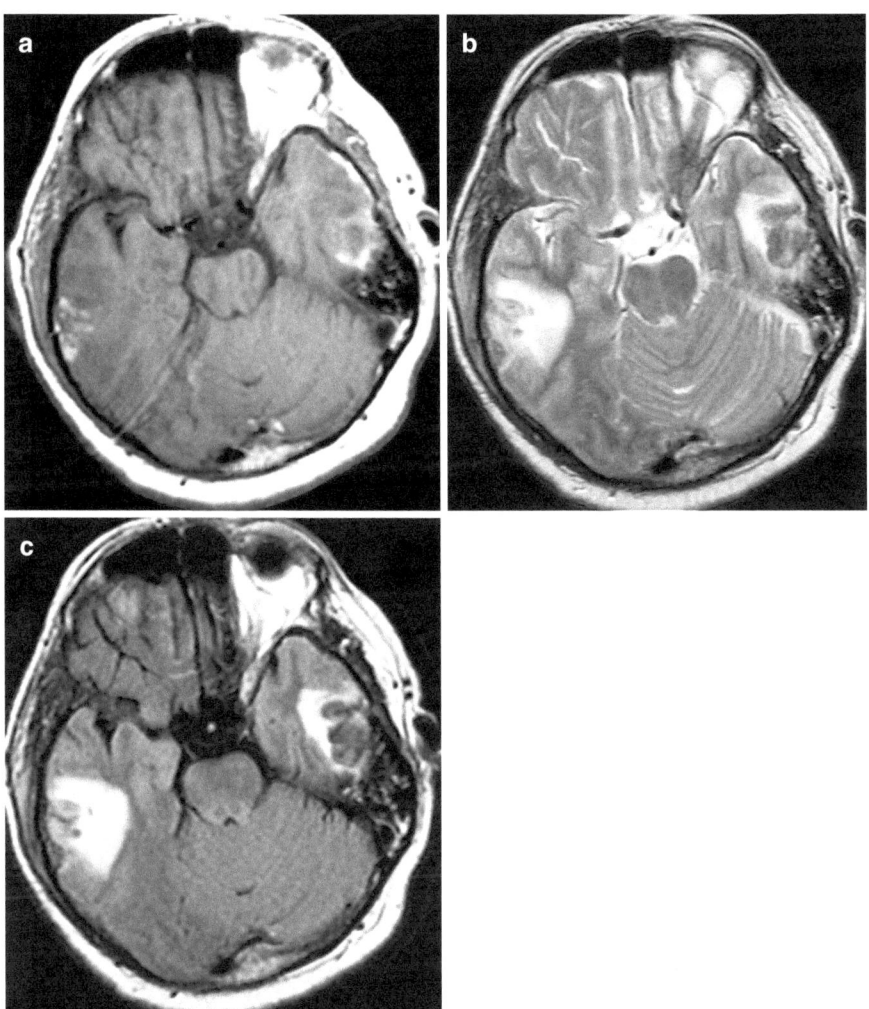

Fig. 3.14 MRI features of supratentorial cortical-subcortical lesions (grade 2 by extended MRI gradation). T1WI (**a**), T2WI (**b**), T2-FLAIR (**c**)

As an example of bilateral injury of the medulla oblongata, we present a case of a patient aged 29 years who got trauma in a motorcycle crash (Fig. 3.20).

In 76 patients of our series, MR examinations detected lesions in the brain stem: 68 (89.5 %) of them were in coma and 58 (76 %) showed unfavorable outcome. Eight patients (10.5 %) of 76 with brain stem lesions were not in coma; their GCS score varied from 9 to 14 (average 12). At the same time, 28 (62.2 %) of 45 patients with MRI signs of deep hemispheric structure injuries (including the thalami, basal ganglia, and corpus callosum and their combinations, excluding brain stem damage) were in coma (GCS ≤ 8), the rest of 16 (37.8 %) in sopor or somnolence (9–14 by GCS).

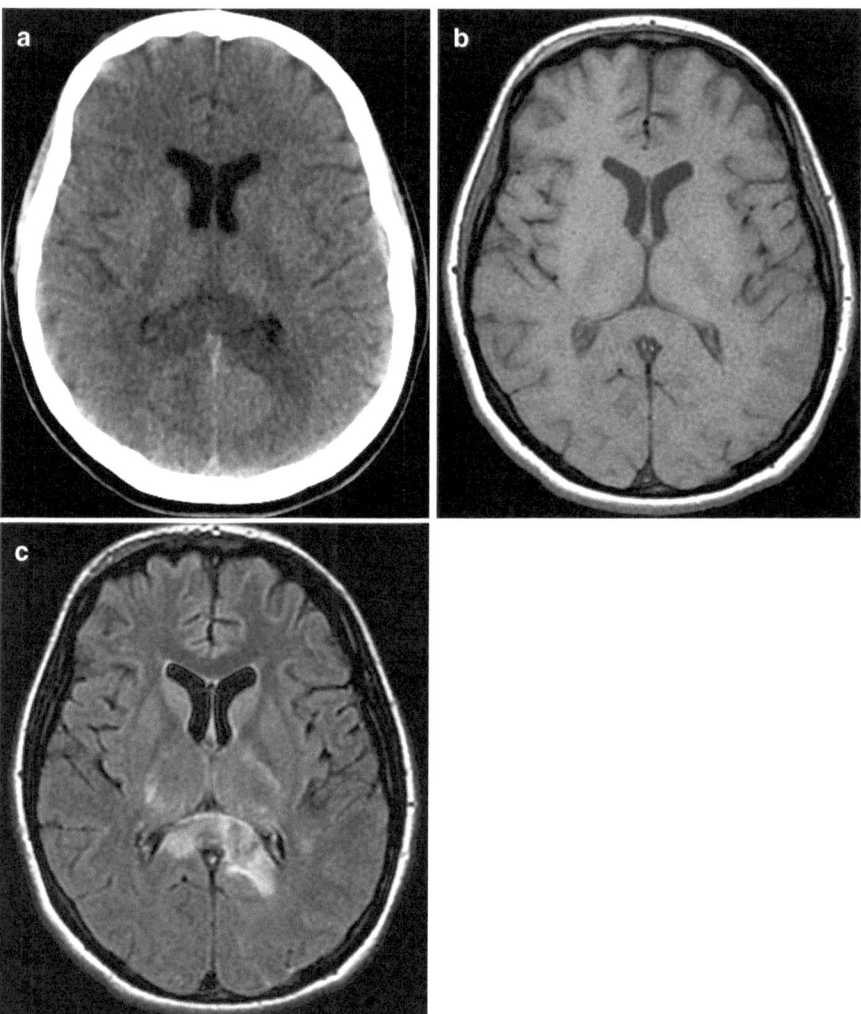

Fig. 3.15 Diffuse axonal injury. GCS, 5. Coma duration, 17 days. Outcome, severe disability. MRI study in 12 days after injury. MR signs of corpus callosum, basal ganglia, and thalamus lesions. Axial CT (**a**) shows a hypodense zone in the splenium of the corpus callosum. Damage area is not visible on T1WI MRI (**b**). T2-FLAIR (**c**) visualized real damaged areas of DAI – the corpus callosum, posterior limb of the internal capsule, and thalamus on the right, posterior limb of the internal capsule and globus pallidus on the left (grade 4 by extended MRI gradation)

Analysis of MRI data showed that brain stem lesion rate increased alongside with TBI severity and reached 80 % in patients in deep coma.

However, brain stem and corpus callosum lesions, i.e., signs of axonal injury, were observed in 2 of 27 patients with mild TBI (GCS 13–15) (Fig. 3.21).

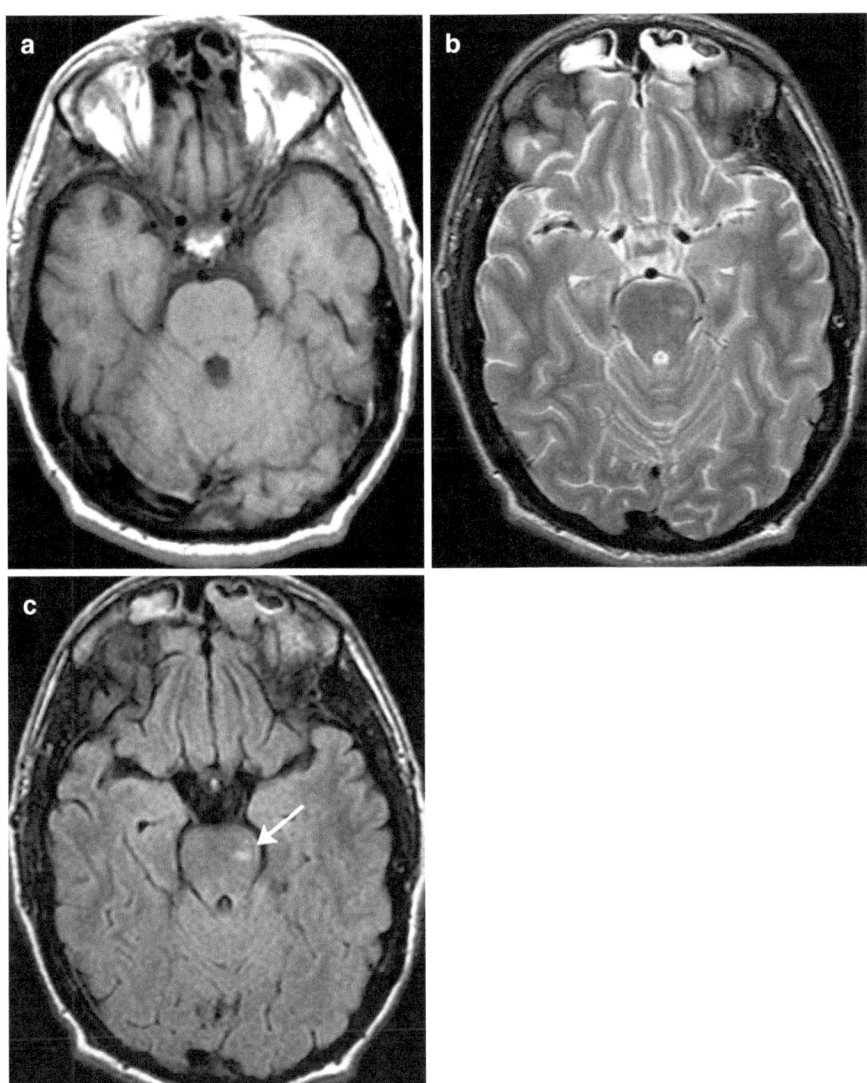

Fig. 3.16 MRI signs of a unilateral damage at the midbrain-pons level on the left (grade 5 by extended MRI gradation). T1WI, (**a**); T2WI, (**b**); T2-FLAIR, (**c**) (*white arrow*)

Case Report (Fig. 3.21)
F., 25 y.o. Traffic accident. Loss of consciousness lasting several minutes, amnesia. Diagnosis: closed head injury, diffuse axonal injury with damages of the corpus callosum, right cerebral peduncle. Right-sided 3rd nerve palsy.

On admission: clear consciousness, GCS score 15. She reveals signs of the right-sided 3rd cranial nerve palsy (dilated and fixed pupil, ptosis, divergent strabismus). Limited temporal extraocular movement (abduction) of the right eye and reduced right corneal reflex are marked.

MRI on the 4th day after trauma: DAI, lesions in the genu and splenium of the corpus callosum. Increased MR signal in T2-FLAIR from medial portions of the right cerebral peduncle.

GOS at discharge: good recovery. Positive dynamics: partial function recovery of the 3d cranial nerve on the right.

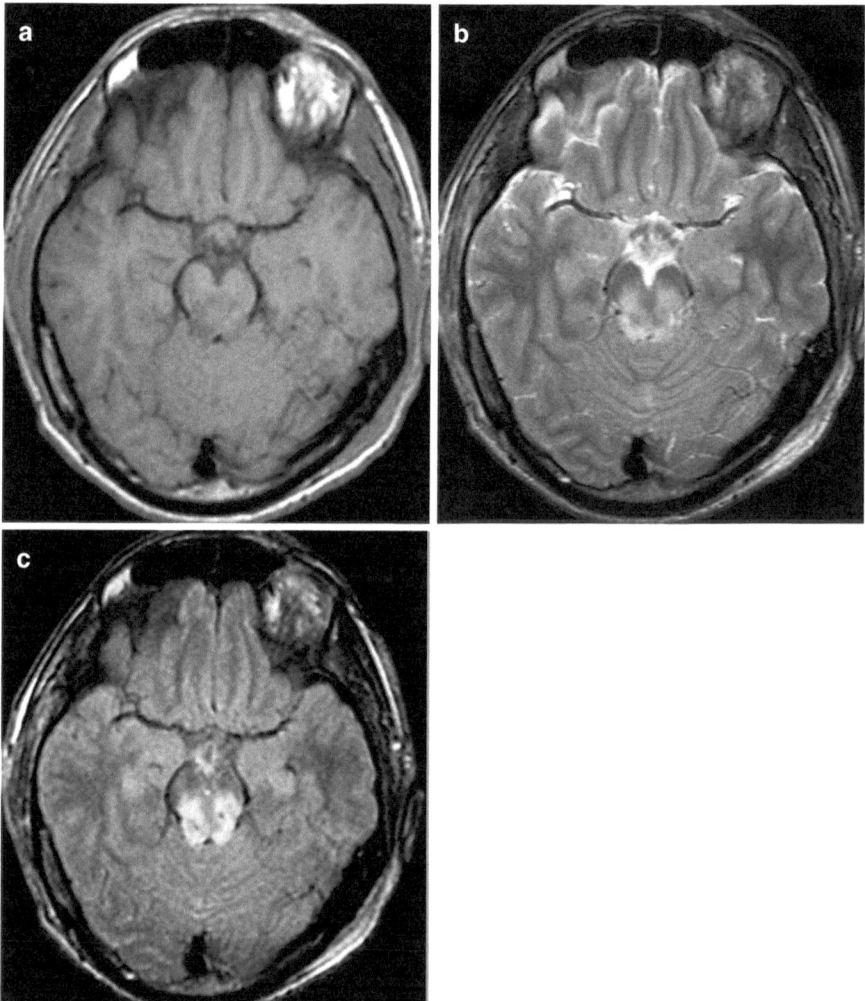

Fig. 3.17 Traffic accident. GCS, 4. Outcome, severe disability. MRI signs of DAI with bilateral damages at the midbrain level (grade 6 by extended MRI gradation). T1WI, (**a**); T2WI, (**b**); T2-FLAIR, (**c**)

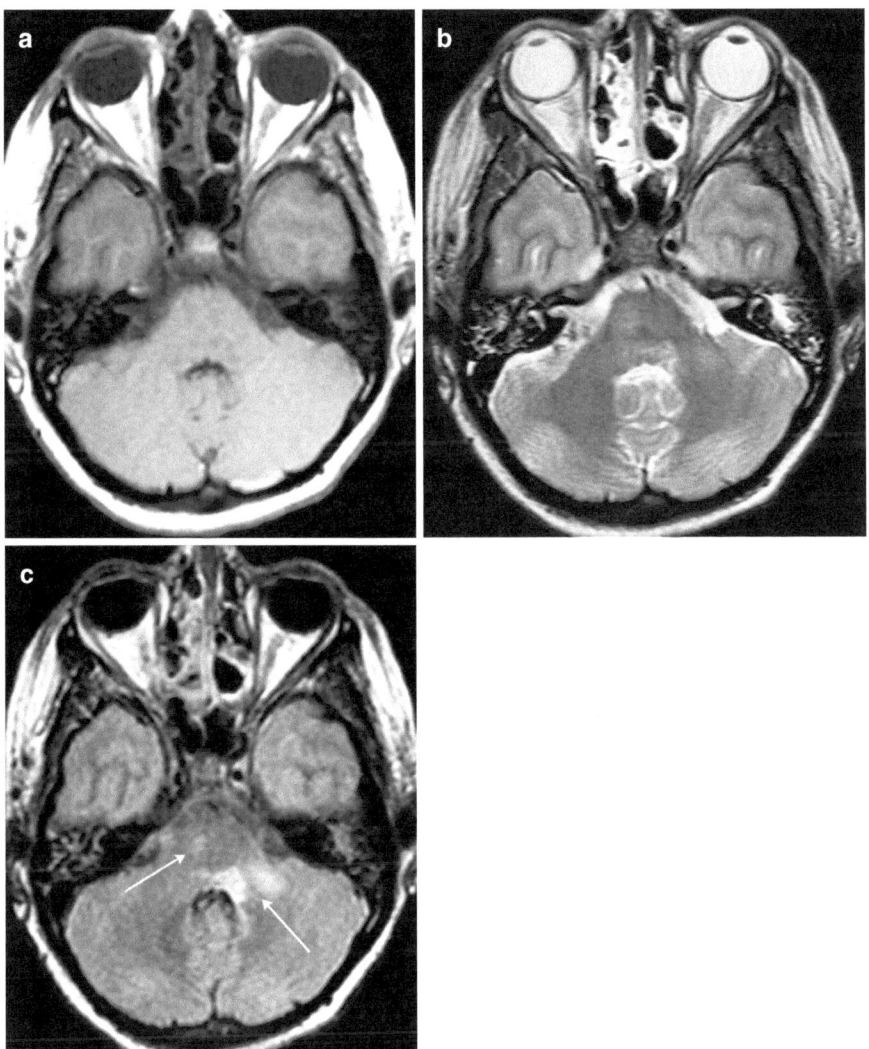

Fig. 3.18 MRI signs of bilateral damages at the pons level (grade 7 by extended MRI gradation). T1WI, (**a**); T2WI, (**b**); T2-FLAIR, (**c**) (*white arrows*)

Having compared our and other authors' data on brain stem injury rate in traumatic coma, we found out some differences in evaluating the severity and time course after TBI, as well as using different MRI sequences (Table 3.10).

As is seen in Table 3.10, brain stem lesion rate in a series of Firsching et al. (2001) made up 57 %, in a series of Mannion et al. (2007) 28 %, and in our series of patients it ranged 49–83 % depending on GCS severity. In our opinion, it may be explained by the use of more sensitive MRI sequences: T2-FLAIR, diffusion-weighted imaging, and gradient echo imaging with high spatial resolution (3D T2* – SWAN) and considerably extended period of examination after injury.

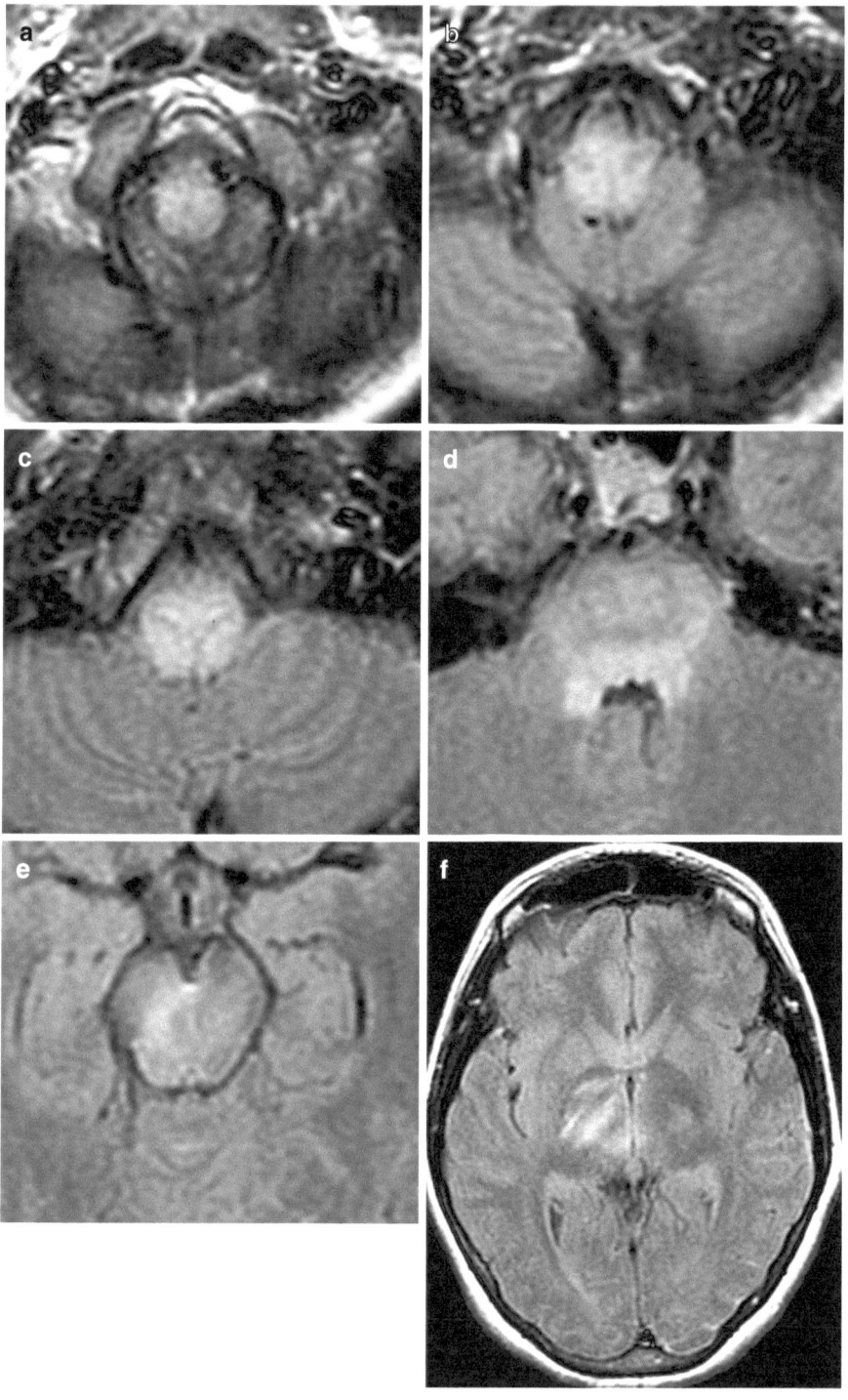

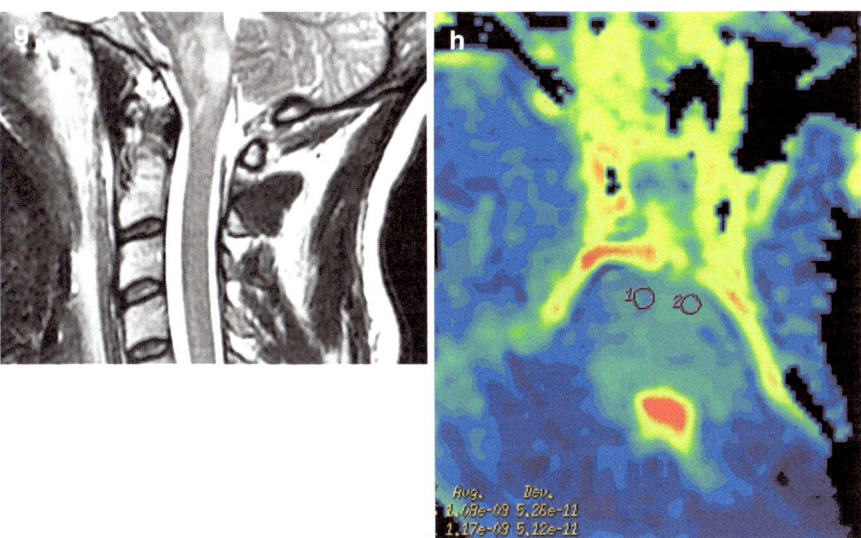

Fig. 3.19 (continued)

The data obtained suggest the extended MRI classification to be highly sensitive for evaluation of severity and location of traumatic brain injury as well as outcome prognosis.

3.3 Discussion

Over the past years the neuroimaging techniques, mainly CT and MRI, have been considerably modified. However, each of them has some advantages and disadvantages, especially in patients with different TBI severity and clinical manifestations. For this reason, new optimal algorithms have been developed and have proved to be essential for making an adequate diagnosis, treatment decisions, as well as outcome prognosis (Haacke et al. 2010).

According to our experience and literature data, neither of the neuroimaging techniques has proved to be absolutely sensitive in detection of all types of acute head trauma and its consequences, as well as evaluation of a wide range of brain and

Fig. 3.19 Traffic accident. Sopor (GCS, 11), episodes of apnea, tetraparesis. MRI in 5 days after trauma (T2-FLAIR, **a–f**; T2WI, **g**) reveals bilateral damages at the levels of the medulla oblongata, pons, and midbrain and also the thalamus and basal ganglia on the right (grade 8 by extended MRI gradation). ADC map (**h**) detects vasogenic edema of the brain stem – 1.08–1.17×10^{-3} mm^2/s (in norm, $0.7 \pm 0.075 \times 10^{-3}$ mm^2/s)

skull pathology in different periods after TBI (Gennarelli et al. 1982; Marshall et al. 1991; Maas et al. 2005; Saatman et al. 2008; Kornienko and Pronin 2009; Potapov et al. 2009). New knowledge about biomechanics, neuromorphology, and pathophysiology of TBI are the basis for its clinical diagnosis of the traumatic brain disease, course, and outcome prognosis.

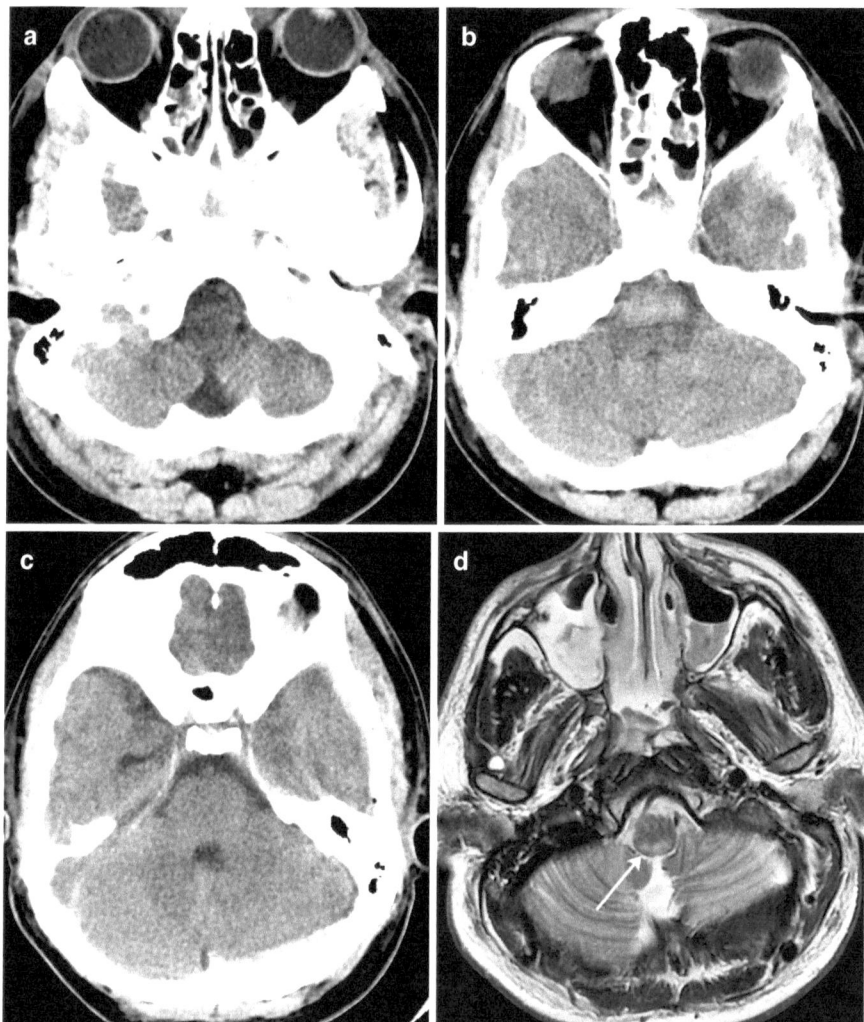

Fig. 3.20 Combined motorcycle trauma. GCS, 7, tetraparesis. Outcome, severe disability, tetraparesis. On admission CT scans (**a–c**) after epidural hematoma removal in the left temporoparietal region, subdural hematoma in the left temporal region, small epidural hematoma (<10 ml) in the posterior fossa on the right. MRI in 4 days after injury (T2WI, **d, e**; T2-FLAIR, **f, g**; DWI, **h, i**) revealed areas of secondary ischemia in different vascular regions and bilateral lesions in the dorsal part of the medulla oblongata (*white arrows*), which was not visualized on CT scans (grade 8 by extended MRI gradation)

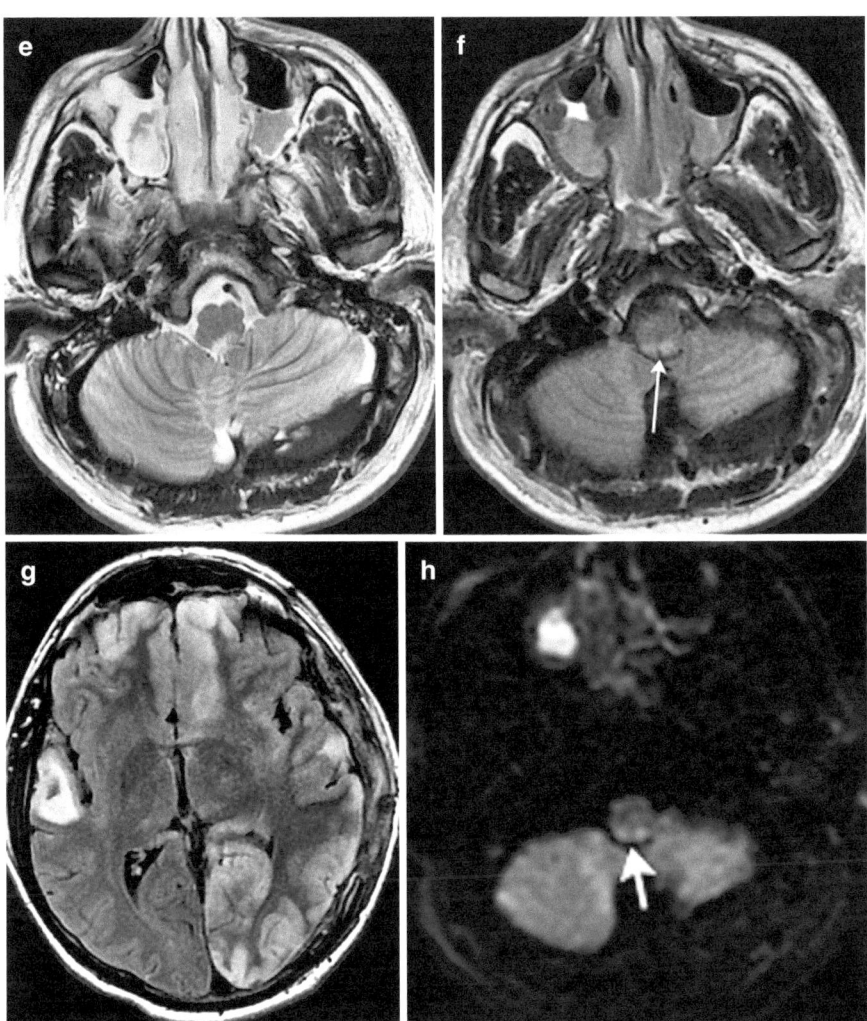

Fig. 3.20 (continued)

Fig. 3.20 (continued)

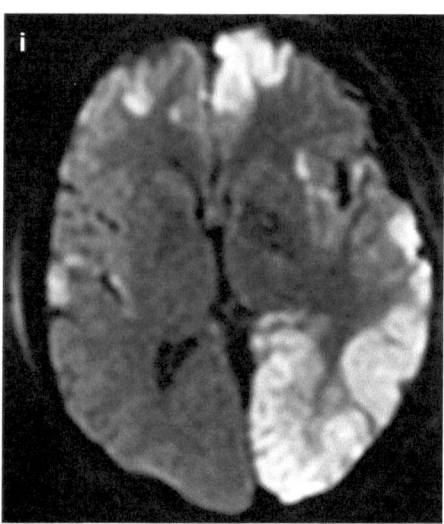

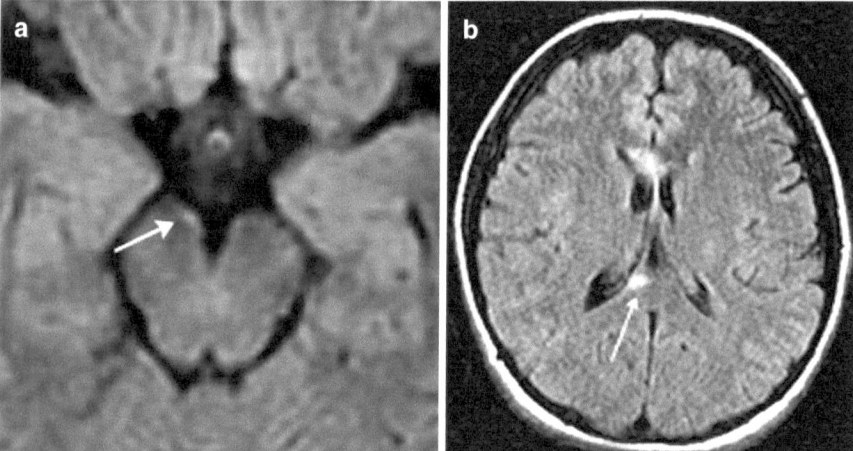

Fig. 3.21 MRI in mild traumatic brain injury. DAI. Traffic accident. Short-term loss of consciousness. GCS, 15. 3rd nerve palsy: ptosis, anisocoria (D > S), divergent strabismus. MRI data: (**a, b**). T2-FLAIR – lesions in the right cerebral peduncle and corpus callosum (*white arrows*)

Proposed MRI grading of hemispheric and brain stem lesions evidently correlated with GCS and GOS. Frequency of coma and unfavorable outcome grow with the involvement of deep hemispheric and brain stem structures.

The data obtained have proved the modern concept that coma in TBI patients results from primary or secondary deep hemispheric (basal ganglia, thalamus) and brain stem structure injury (Levin 2006; Schiff 2008, 2009). Besides, MRI allowed

Table 3.10 Brain stem injury rate in comatose patients (GCS ≤ 8) after TBI by our data ($n = 106$) and other authors

	Our data, GCS 3–4	Our data, GCS 5–6	Our data, GCS 7–8	Firsching et al. (2001), GCS < 8	Mannion et al. (2007), GCS < 9 (*)
MRI sequences	T1,T2, T2-FLAIR, DWI, GRE	T1,T2, T2-FLAIR, DWI, GRE	T1,T2, T2-FLAIR, DWI, GRE	T1,T2	T1, T2, FLAIR, GRE
Days after injury	≤21	≤21	≤21	≤8	≤4
Total (n)	23	38	45	102	46
Brain stem injury (%)	83	68	49	57	28

*Authors indicated that all patients had severe TBI and all of them were intubated and ventilated for more than 24 h

detecting brain stem injuries at a higher rate in comatose patients in our group compared to those with the data published earlier (Marshall et al. 1991; Firsching et al. 2001; Saatman et al. 2008; Lagares et al. 2009; Hilario et al. 2012).

Our results have supported other authors' conclusions that incidence of coma is evidently higher for brain stem injuries compared to supratentorial hemispheric injuries. However, primary brain stem injuries including the midbrain, pons, and even medulla oblongata may be revealed in patients with a conscious level ranging from obnubilation to sopor with further consciousness recovery. These data are consistent with studies of other authors (Bazarian et al. 2007; Haacke et al. 2010) and show that some MRI sequences (SWAN, DWI, DTI) are more sensitive in detecting nonhemorrhagic damage of the basal ganglia, corpus callosum, and brain stem in moderate and even mild head injuries.

By using this approach we found out that traffic accidents proved to be the most frequent cause of damage to deep brain structures compared to other causes of trauma.

These data confirm the concept that traffic accidents are the main cause of DAI because deep brain structure injury is typical for this type of TBI.

The developed extended MRI classification revealed statistically significant correlations with trauma severity, as well as outcome.

Thus, today, a new data on the anatomy of brain trauma of different severity has been accumulated due to an introduction into clinical practice and widespread of modern highly sensitive neuroimaging technologies. Therefore, there is a strong necessity for new revisions and renovations of the existing classifications which will allow evaluating a wide spectrum of clinical and morphological manifestations of neurotrauma depending on different mechanisms and other factors like premorbidity, age, gender, etc. The proposed extended MRI classification of the brain injury location and level can serve as an example of efficacy of this approach. Further studies of TBI neuroimaging will open up new vistas for outlining a modern, advanced prognostic model of neurotrauma and developing a new clinical and morphological classification of TBI.

References

Alexandrova E, Zaitsev O, Tenedieva V, Potapov A, Zakharova N et al (2011) Plasma catecholamines in consciousness recovery in patients with severe traumatic brain injury. Zh Neurol Psikhiatr im SSKorsakova 3:58–63

Augustenborg CC (2010) Endogenous feedback network: a new approach to the comprehensive study of consciousness. Conscious cognit 19:547–579

Bazarian J, Zhong J, Blyth B et al (2007) Diffusion tensor imaging detects clinically important axonal damage after mild traumatic brain injury: a pilot study. J Neurotrauma 24:1447–1459

Bragina N, Potapov A, Zaitsev O, Zakharova N et al (2011) Predominant brain lesion level. In: Zaitsev O (ed) Psychopathology of severe head injury. MEDpressinform, Moscow, pp 226–236

Castaigne P et al (1981) Paramedian thalamic and midbrain infarcts: clinical and neuropathological study. Ann Neurol 10:127–148

Firsching R, Woischneck D, Klein S et al (2001) Classification of severe head injury based on magnetic resonance imaging. Acta Neurochir 143:263–271

Gennarelli T, Thibault L, Adams J et al (1982) Diffuse axonal injury and traumatic coma in the primate. Ann Neurol 12:564–574

Haacke E, Duhaime A, Gean A et al (2010) Common data elements in radiologic imaging of traumatic brain injury. J Magn Reson Imaging 32(3):516–543

Hilario A, Ramos A, Millan JM et al (2012) Severe traumatic head injury: prognostic value of brain stem injuries detected at MRI. AJNR Am J Neuroradiol 33:1925–1931

Kornienko V, Pronin I (eds) (2009) Diagnostic neuroradiology. Springer, Berlin/Heidelberg

Lagares A, Ramos A, Derez-Nunes A et al (2009) The role of MRI in assessing prognosis after severe and moderate head injury. Acta Neurochir 151:341–356

Lammi M et al (2005) The minimally conscious state and recovery potential: a follow-up study 2 to 5 years after traumatic brain injury. Arch Phys Med Rehabil 86:746–754

Levin B (2006) Introduction to neuroimaging in traumatic brain injury. J Neurotrauma 23(10): 1394–1396

Maas A, Hukkelhoven C, Marshall L et al (2005) Prediction of outcome in traumatic brain injury with computed tomographic characteristics a comparison between the computed tomographic classification and combinations of computed tomographic predictors. Neurosurgery 57:1173–1182

Mannion R, Cross J, Bradley P et al (2007) Mechanism-based MRI classification of traumatic brainstem injury and its relationship to outcome. J Neurotrauma 24:128–135

Marshall L, Marshall S, Klauber M, Clark M (1991) A new classification of head injury based on computerized tomography. J Neurosurg 75:14–20

Maxwell W (2006) Thalamic nuclei after human blunt head injury. J Neuropathol Exp Neurol 65:478–488

McMillan T, Herbert C (2004) Further recovery in a potential treatment withdrawal case 10 years after brain injury. Brain Inj 18:935–940

Munkle MC et al (2000) The distribution of calbindin, calretinin and parvalbumin immunoreactivity in the human thalamus. J Chem Neuroanat 19:155–173

Oknina L, Sharova E, Zaitsev O, Zakharova N, Masherov E, Schekutiev G, Kornienko V, Potapov A (2011) Long-latency components (N100, N200 and P300) of acoustic evoked potentials in prediction of mental recovery in severe traumatic brain injury. Zh Vopr Neurokhir im NNBurdenko 75(3):19–30

Owen AM et al (2006) Detecting awareness in the vegetative state. Science 313:1402

Posner J, Saper C, Schiff N, Plum F (2007) Plum and posner's diagnosis of stupor and coma. In: Plum F, Posner J (eds) 4th edn. Oxford University Press, New York

Potapov A, Likhterman L (2011) Management of severe traumatic brain injuries. In: Kalangu K, Kato Y, Dechambinoit G (eds) Essential practice of neurosurgery. WFNS/Asses Publishing Co Ltd, Japan

Potapov A, Kravchuk A, Zakharova N (2009) Head trauma. In: Kornienko V, Pronin I (eds) Diagnostic neuroradiology. Springer, Heidelberg, pp 807–919

Saatman K, Duhaime A, Bullock R et al (2008) Classification of traumatic brain injury for targeted therapies. J Neurotrauma 25:719–728

Schiff N (2008) Central thalamic contributions to arousal regulation and neurological disorders of consciousness. Ann N Y Acad Sci 1129:105–118

Schiff N (2009) Recovery of consciousness after brain injury: a mesocircuit hypothesis. Trends Neurosci 33(1):1–9

Schiff N, Plum F (2000) The role of arousal and 'gating' systems in the neurology of impaired consciousness. J Clin Neurophysiol 17:438–452

Dynamic Study of White Matter Fiber Tracts After Traumatic Brain Injury

4

Contents

4.1 Quantitative Evaluation of Corpus Callosum and Corticospinal Tract Condition
in the Acute Period of TBI.. 69
4.2 Dynamic DT-MRI Study of Corpus Callosum and Corticospinal Tracts 74
4.3 Discussion 102
References.. 105

4.1 Quantitative Evaluation of Corpus Callosum and Corticospinal Tract Condition in the Acute Period of TBI

Quantitative DT-MRI analysis was performed in 22 patients aged 9–54 years (average 25 years, 13 males, 11 females) and in 8 healthy volunteers (control group) aged 22–57 years (average 33 years, 5 males, 3 females). All 22 patients were in coma (GCS of 4–8, average 6) on admission to the Burdenko Neurosurgery Institute, which lasted 3–20 days (average 12 days). CT revealed signs of DAI in all patients (categories I–IV according to Marshall et al. 1991). The outcomes in 3 months after injury in the analyzed group were as follows: good recovery in 3 patients, moderate disability in 7, severe disability in 9, and vegetative state in 3. MRI studies for these 22 patients were performed within 2–17 days of TBI, average of 10 days. The selection criteria for MRI studies were as follows: stabilization of patient's condition, normalization of intracranial pressure and hemodynamics, adequate ventilation, and absence of metallic implants.

No statistically significant differences were found in ADC and FA between the right and left sides in the control group (Table 4.1). For this reason, all bilateral measurements in the control subjects were averaged.

At the same time, average FA values in the control group along the corticospinal tracts at the level of pons were significantly lower compared to cerebral peduncles and internal capsule (Fig. 4.1).

Table 4.1 Average ADC and FA values for the control group

ROI	ADC values × 10^{-3} ± SD × 10^{-3}, mm²/s		
	Right	Left	*p*-value
CST at the level:			
PLIC	0.699 ± 0.05	0.716 ± 0.05	0.489
Midbrain	0.779 ± 0.03	0.799 ± 0.09	0.571
Pons	0.732 ± 0.1	0.711 ± 0.1	0.673
Genu of CC	0.852 ± 0.069	0.857 ± 0.07	0.885
Splenium of CC	0.791 ± 0.1	0.789 ± 0.1	0.973
	FA values ± SD		
	Right	Left	*p*-value
CST at the level:			
PLIC	0.714 ± 0.02	0.695 ± 0.02	0.081
Midbrain	0.717 ± 0.038	0.698 ± 0.049	0.451
Pons	0.573 ± 0.04	0.553 ± 0.04	0.317
Genu of CC	0.755 ± 0.045	0.739 ± 0.045	0.526
Splenium of CC	0.787 ± 0.051	0.786 ± 0.051	0.965

ROI region of interest, *CST* corticospinal tract, *PLIC* posterior limb of the internal capsule, *CC* corpus callosum, *SD* standard deviation

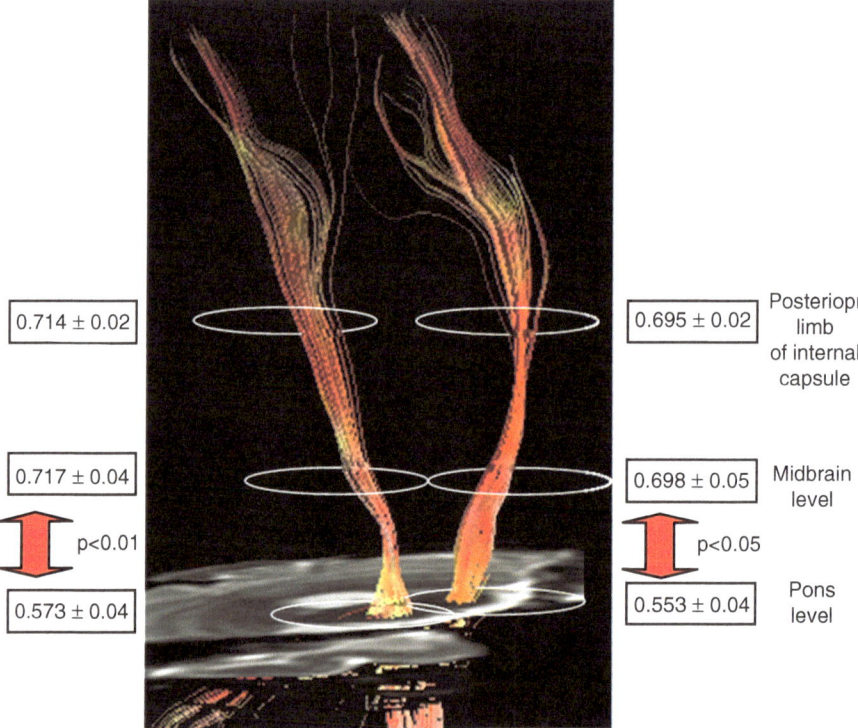

Fig. 4.1 Average fractional anisotropy values alongside the corticospinal tracts in healthy volunteers

Table 4.2 Comparison of bilateral average ADC and FA values in patients without paresis ($n=7$)

ROI	ADC values $\times 10^{-3} \pm$ SD $\times 10^{-3}$, mm²/s		
	Right	Left	*p*-value
CST:			
PLIC	0.732±0.047	0.761±0.139	0.471
Midbrain	0.761±0.074	0.749±0.09	0.75
Pons	0.756±0.06	0.724±0.084	0.308
ROI	FA values ± SD		
	Right	Left	*p*-value
CST:			
PLIC	0.638±0.106	0.652±0.125	0.764
Midbrain	0.622±0.114	0.629±0.085	0.857
Pons	0.515±0.085	0.501±0.082	0.696

ROI region of interest, *CST* corticospinal tract, *PLIC* posterior limb of the internal capsule, *SD* standard deviation

Table 4.3 Comparison of averaged ADC and FA values in patients without paresis ($n=7$) and in control group ($n=8$)

ROI	ADC values $\times 10^{-3} \pm$ SD $\times 10^{-3}$, mm²/s		
	Control group	Patients	*p*-value
CST:			
PLIC	0.708±0.047	0.743±0.092	0.071
Midbrain	0.789±0.063	0.756±0.08	0.066
Pons	0.722±0.1	0.744±0.07	0.131
ROI	FA values ± SD		
	Control group	Patients	*p*-value
CST:			
PLIC	0.704±0.02	0.643±0.111	0.041
Midbrain	0.708±0.044	0.625±0.101	0.0007
Pons	0.563±0.04	0.510±0.082	0.013

ROI region of interest, *CST* corticospinal tract, *PLIC* posterior limb of internal capsule, *SD* standard deviation

The results of comparisons of bilateral ADC and FA values in seven patients without paresis are presented in Table 4.2.

Table 4.2 shows that no statistically significant differences were noted for ADC and FA between the right and left sides along corticospinal tracts in patients without motor disturbances. Thus, they were also averaged. The average ADC and average FA values in this group were compared with those in the control group (Table 4.3).

There was a statistically significant FA value reduction along the corticospinal tracts in patients without hemiparesis compared with the control group, but no differences were observed for ADC values in any region (Table 4.3).

A statistically significant FA reduction was found at the cerebral peduncle level ($p<0.05$) in the homolateral to hemiparesis CST in patients with hemiparesis ($n=11$) compared to the control group (Table 4.4).

Table 4.4 Comparison of averaged ADC and FA values in homolateral to hemiparesis side in patients ($n=11$) and in control group ($n=8$)

ROI	ADC values × 10^{-3} ± SD × 10^{-3}, mm²/s		
	Control group	Patients	p-value
CST:			
PLIC	0.708 ± 0.047	0.733 ± 0.049	0.088
Midbrain	0.789 ± 0.063	0.785 ± 0.079	0.444
Pons	0.722 ± 0.1	0.749 ± 0.101	0.249
ROI	FA values ± SD		
	Control group	Patients	p-value
CST:			
PLIC	0.704 ± 0.02	0.677 ± 0.092	0.296
Midbrain	0.708 ± 0.044	0.666 ± 0.068	0.034
Pons	0.563 ± 0.04	0.528 ± 0.111	0.192

ROI region of interest, *CST* corticospinal tract, *PLIC* posterior limb of the internal capsule, *SD* standard deviation

Table 4.5 Comparison of averaged ADC and FA values in contralateral to hemiparesis side ($n=11$) and in control group ($n=8$)

ROI	ADC values × 10^{-3} ± SD × 10^{-3}, mm²/s		
	Control group	Patients	p-value
CST:			
PLIC	0.708 ± 0.047	0.785 ± 0.116	0.011
Midbrain	0.789 ± 0.063	0.786 ± 0.055	0.450
Pons	0.722 ± 0.1	0.753 ± 0.085	0.198
ROI	FA values ± SD		
	Control group	Patients	p-value
CST:			
PLIC	0.704 ± 0.02	0.590 ± 0.136	0.0065
Midbrain	0.708 ± 0.044	0.585 ± 0.126	0.0011
Pons	0.563 ± 0.04	0.509 ± 0.096	0.055

ROI region of interest, *CST* corticospinal tract, *PLIC* posterior limb of the internal capsule, *SD* standard deviation

Statistically significant differences were observed for FA in the posterior limb of the internal capsule (PLIC) and peduncles and for ADC in PLIC on the contralateral to hemiparesis side of CST in patients with hemiparesis compared to the control group (Table 4.5).

A statistically significant difference in FA values was found in the cerebral peduncles and PLIC between homolateral and contralateral sides in patients with hemiparesis (Table 4.6, Fig. 4.2).

A statistically significant FA reduction was noted in all regions of interest along the CSTs when comparing 4 patients with tetraparesis to the control group (Table 4.7).

The study showed that FA values in the corpus callosum and along the corticospinal tracts as well as ADC values in the splenium of the corpus callosum significantly correlated ($p<0.01$) with outcome in patients examined within 10–17 days after TBI (Table 4.8). However, there was no significant correlation between clinical outcome and diffusion parameters when patients were scanned 2–9 days following trauma.

Table 4.6 Comparison of averaged ADC and FA values in homo- and contralateral sides in 11 patients with hemiparesis

ROI	ADC values × 10^{-3} ± SD × 10^{-3}, mm²/s		
	Homolateral	Contralateral	*p*-value
CST:			
PLIC	0.733 ± 0.049	0.785 ± 0.116	0.092
Midbrain	0.785 ± 0.079	0.786 ± 0.055	0.486
Pons	0.749 ± 0.101	0.753 ± 0.085	0.460
ROI	FA values ± SD		
	Homolateral	Contralateral	*p*-value
CST:			
PLIC	0.677 ± 0.092	0.590 ± 0.136	0.046
Midbrain	0.666 ± 0.068	0.585 ± 0.126	0.036
Pons	0.528 ± 0.111	0.509 ± 0.096	0.355

ROI region of interest, *CST* corticospinal tract, *PLIC* posterior limb of the internal capsule, *SD* standard deviation

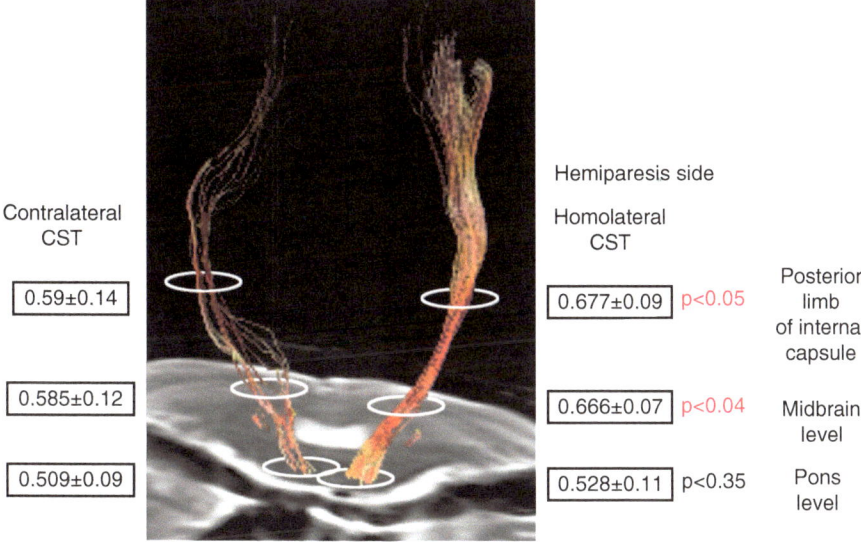

Fig. 4.2 Average fractional anisotropy values alongside the corticospinal tracts in patients with hemiparesis

Comparisons of average ADC and FA values for the genu and splenium of the corpus callosum were performed in all groups of patients with DAI: with no paresis (7), with unilateral paresis (11), with tetraparesis (4), and in control group (8) (Table 4.9).

As can be seen from Table 4.9, all patients, as well as those divided into three subgroups (without paresis, hemi- and tetraparesis) demonstrated an average FA to be significantly lower in the genu and splenium compared to the control group ($p < 0.01$) (Fig. 4.3). Average ADC values in the splenium were significantly lower for all patients compared with control group, thus suggesting a cytotoxic edema (Potapov et al. 2009). Average ADC values in the genu and splenium of the corpus callosum in

Table 4.7 Comparison of averaged ADC and FA values in patients with tetraparesis ($n=4$) and in control group ($n=8$)

ROI	ADC values $\times 10^{-3} \pm SD \times 10^{-3}$, mm²/s		
	Control group	Patients	*p*-value
CST:			
PLIC	0.708 ± 0.047	0.699 ± 0.057	0.165
Midbrain	0.789 ± 0.063	0.793 ± 0.094	0.704
Pons	0.722 ± 0.1	0.668 ± 0.158	0.002
ROI	FA values ± SD		
	Control group	Patients	*p*-value
CST:			
PLIC	0.704 ± 0.02	0.634 ± 0.071	<0.00001
Midbrain	0.708 ± 0.044	0.579 ± 0.151	<0.00001
Pons	0.563 ± 0.04	0.477 ± 0.076	<0.00001

ROI region of interest, *CST* corticospinal tract, *PLIC* posterior limb of the internal capsule, *SD* standard deviation

Table 4.8 Correlation between averaged ADC and FA values and outcome (by GOS) in patients examined within 10–17 days after injury

ADC values	R-value (Correlation coefficient)	*p*-value
PLIC	−0.068	0.749
Midbrain	−0.167	0.435
Pons	−0.213	0.317
Genu of CC	−0.141	0.512
Splenium of CC	−0.512	0.010
FA values	R-value (Correlation coefficient)	*p*-value
PLIC	0.660	0.0004
Midbrain	0.390	0.059
Pons	0.635	0.0008
Genu of CC	0.534	0.007
Splenium of CC	0.415	0.044

ROI region of interest, *PLIC* posterior limb of the internal capsule, *CC* corpus callosum, *SD* standard deviation

patients without paresis were lower than in the control group, but not statistically significant. We revealed a significant decrease of ADC values only in the splenium in patients with hemiparesis. A statistically evident increase in ADC was found in the genu of CC in patients with tetraparesis and thus suggesting a vasogenic edema.

4.2   Dynamic DT-MRI Study of Corpus Callosum and Corticospinal Tracts

Twenty-two patients were examined in dynamics for a qualitative analysis of fiber structures. It was found that only 4 of 22 patients after an 8–15-day coma reached favorable outcome 3 months after injury: good recovery was observed in 1 patient,

Table 4.9 Comparison of averaged ADC and FA values in the genu and splenium of the corpus callosum in patients with diffuse axonal injury and in control group

ROI	ADC values × 10^{-3} ± SD × 10^{-3}, mm^2/s		
	Control group	Without paresis	*p*-value
Genu of CC	0.855±0.067	0.847±0.226	0.449
Splenium of CC	0.790±0.098	0.698±0.092	0.0681
	FA values ± SD		
	Control group	Without paresis	*p*-value
Genu of CC	0.748±0.044	0.655±0.075	0.0046
Splenium of CC	0.786±0.049	0.639±0.119	0.007
	ADC values × 10^{-3} ± SD × 10^{-3}, mm^2/s		
	Control group	Hemiparesis	*p*-value
Genu of CC	0.855±0.067	0.903±0.158	0.081
Splenium of CC	0.790±0.098	0.681±0.148	0.018
	FA values ± SD		
	Control group	Hemiparesis	*p*-value
Genu of CC	0.748±0.044	0.625±0.129	0.001
Splenium of CC	0.786±0.049	0.604±0.128	0.0001
	ADC values × 10^{-3} ± SD × 10^{-3}, mm^2/s		
	Control group	Tetraparesis	*p*-value
Genu of CC	0.855±0.067	0.948±0.098	0.023
Splenium of CC	0.790±0.098	0.700±0.226	0.159
	FA values ± SD		
	Control group	Tetraparesis	*p*-value
Genu of CC	0.748±0.044	0.607±0.090	0.0003
Splenium of CC	0.786±0.049	0.532±0.171	0.0003
	ADC values × 10^{-3} ± SD × 10^{-3}, mm^2/s		
	Control group	All patients	*p*-value
Genu of CC	0.855±0.067	0.892±0.156	0.287
Splenium of CC	0.790±0.098	0.710±0.137	0.034
	FA values ± SD		
	Control group	All patients	*p*-value
Genu of CC	0.748±0.044	0.656±0.115	0.0007
Splenium of CC	0.786±0.049	0.643±0.142	0.0001

ROI region of interest, *CC* corpus callosum, *SD* standard deviation

and moderate disability with no serious signs of mental, motor, and sensory disturbances was observed in the remaining three (Table 4.10). Fifteen patients after coma lasting 3–20 days were severely disabled in 3 months after trauma due to transient or persistent mental disturbances. Thirteen of them were known to have severe motor impairment in the form of hemiparesis ($n = 7$) or tetraparesis ($n = 6$). Three months after injury 3 of 22 patients after a 14–22-day coma were in the vegetative state with signs of tetraparesis (Table 4.10, case reports 13, 14, 20). One of them died after being in vegetative state for 7 months, one remained in a persistent vegetative state, and the other one emerged from the vegetative state, but was found to be severely disabled (minimally conscious state, aphasia, tetraparesis) in 3 years later.

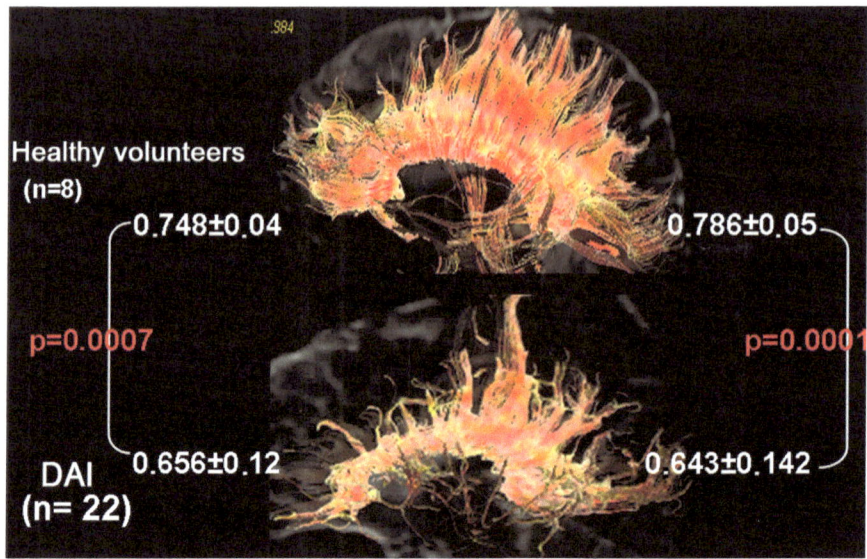

Fig. 4.3 Average FA values in the corpus callosum in healthy volunteers and patients in the acute stage of DAI

Primary MRI scan performed within 2–21 days after injury showed that 4 of 22 patients had only hemispheric injuries; 18 patients had signs of brain stem damage at the midbrain level ($n=16$) and at the level of the pons ($n=2$) along with hemispheric lesions (Table 4.10).

Repeated DTI was performed in 9 patients, within 4–9 weeks after injury, and in 13 patients, within 3–36 months following trauma; in 3 of 22 cases DTI was repeated 3 times and more.

Qualitative analysis of the initial DT-MRI with 3D reconstructions of brain pathways performed 2–22 days after injury showed that the CC in 4 patients and CST in 5 patients did not differ from controls (Fig. 4.4). Normally appearing three-dimensional structures of the CC and CST in the first study were observed in both patients with favorable outcome and those whose condition resulted in severe disability.

The structure of the CC in 3 patients remained normal 1 month after trauma; however, one of them showed good recovery; the second had moderate disability and the third severe disability. Three years later the third patient showed moderate disability (Table 4.10, patient 7).

Repeated examination of 12 patients at different time following injury (with coma lasting from 3 to 17 days) revealed a reduction in the "density" or shortening of fibers extending from the CC (mainly in frontal and occipital regions) accompanied by partial atrophy (Table 4.10, Fig. 4.5).

Three months post-injury 10 of 12 patients remained profoundly disabled with mental and neurological disorders. Two patients recovered to moderate disability.

Table 4.10 Main characteristics of analyzed patients

N	Age, gender	GCS	Coma duration (days)	MRI data: brain stem injury	MRI data: corticospinal tracts	MRI data: corpus callosum	Clinical data	GOS in 3 months	GOS >3 months
1	24, m	5	8	–	Norm	Norm	Orientation recovery by day 32 after injury, regression of moderate right-sided hemiparesis	Good recovery	
2	19, f	5	15	+	Asymmetry, worse on the right side	Norm	Orientation recovery by day 39, dysarthria, mild left-sided hemiparesis, ataxia	Moderate disability	
3	9, f	6	3	+	Absent on the right side, thinning on the left side	Partial atrophy	Orientation recovery by day 36 after trauma, severe left-sided hemiparesis	Severe disability	
4	30, f	5	7	–	Norm	Partial atrophy	By month 1: obeys commands, amnestic confusion for 3 months, cognitive and personality disorders, no motor deficit	Severe disability	In 3 years: moderate disability
5	23, f	5	9	+	Asymmetry, worse on the right side	Partial atrophy	Orientation recovery after 2.5 months, cognitive and personality disorders, severe left-sided hemiparesis	Severe disability	In 6 months: severe disability, left-sided hemiparesis
6	14, f	6	10	–	Norm	Partial atrophy	Orientation recovery after 3 months after trauma, no paresis	Severe disability	

(continued)

Table 4.10 (continued)

N	Age, gender	GCS	Coma duration (days)	MRI data: brain stem injury	MRI data: corticospinal tracts	MRI data: corpus callosum	Clinical data	GOS in 3 months	GOS >3 months
7	34, m	4	20	+	Asymmetry, worse on the right side	Norm	After 1 month: obeys commands, orientation recovery after 3 months, regression of left-sided hemiparesis in 1 year	Severe disability	In 3 years: moderate disability
8	29, f	6	6	+	Asymmetry, worse on the left side	Partial atrophy	After 1 month: speech comprehension, after 2 months: speech attempt, after 3 months: orientation recovery Severe right-sided hemiparesis	Severe disability	In 3 years: severe disability, right-sided hemiparesis
9	20, f	5	17	+	Bilateral thinning, worse on the right side	Partial atrophy	Duration of unconsciousness state over 2 months, mutism, speech comprehension after 2.5 months, tetraparesis	Severe disability	In 4 years: severe disability, left-sided hemiparesis
10	22, f	4	17	+	Asymmetry, worse on the left side	Total atrophy	Duration of unconsciousness state for 42 days after trauma. In 3 months: aphasia, tetraparesis	Severe disability	In 8 months: severe disability, tetraparesis
11	35, m	5	16	+	Asymmetry, worse on the right side	Total atrophy	Speech comprehension from day 32, speech attempt from day 61, further – Korsakoff's syndrome over 10 months. Tetraparesis deeper on the left side	Severe disability	In 1 year: severe disability, tetraparesis

12	41, m	7	14	+	Bilateral thinning, worse on the right side	Total atrophy	Vegetative state for more than 2 months After 4 months: speech attempt after 1 year: incomplete contact, tetraparesis	Severe disability	In 1 year: severe disability, tetraparesis
13	34, m	5	8	+	Bilateral thinning	Total atrophy	Vegetative state for 2 months with further minimally conscious state, tetraparesis, epilepsy	Vegetative state	In 3 years: minimally conscious state, tetraparesis
14	39, m	6	14	+	Bilateral thinning	Total atrophy	Persistent vegetative state, tetraparesis Death in 7 months	Vegetative state	In 7 months: vegetative state → death
15	22, m	5	10	+	Bilateral thinning, worse on the right side	Partial atrophy	Orientation recovery by day 21, regression of moderate right-sided hemiparesis	Moderate disability	In 6 months: moderate disability, mild left-sided hemiparesis
16	17, f	8	5	+	Asymmetry, worse on the right side	Partial atrophy	Orientation recovery in 16 days, left-sided hemiparesis	Severe disability	In 3 years: moderate disability, mild left-sided hemiparesis
17	23, m	5	14	+	Bilateral thinning, worse on the right side	Partial atrophy	Orientation recovery by day 45, tetraparesis	Severe disability, tetraparesis	In 3 years: moderate disability, mild left-sided hemiparesis

(continued)

Table 4.10 (continued)

N	Age, gender	GCS	Coma duration (days)	MRI data: brain stem injury	MRI data: corticospinal tracts	MRI data: corpus callosum	Clinical data	GOS in 3 months	GOS >3 months
18	35, f	5	10	+	Asymmetry, worse on the right side	Partial atrophy	By day 27, mutism with speech comprehension After 3 months: cognitive and personality disorders, left-sided hemiparesis	Severe disability	In 9 months: severe disability, left-sided hemiparesis
19	17, f	7	10	–	Mild asymmetry, worse on the right side	Partial atrophy	Full consciousness recovery by day 25, regression of left-sided hemiparesis	Moderate disability	In 6 months: moderate disability, mild left-sided hemiparesis
20	72, f	4	22	+	Bilateral thinning	Total atrophy	By day 14: emerging from coma into persistent vegetative state, tetraparesis	Vegetative state	In 16 months: vegetative state, tetraparesis
21	18, f	4	6	+	Bilateral thinning, worse on the right side	Total atrophy	Orientation recovery after 4 months, cognitive and personality disorders, tetraparesis	Severe disability, tetraparesis	In 10 months: severe disability, left-sided hemiparesis
22	26, m	5	8	+	Asymmetry, worse on the left side	Partial atrophy	By day 22: emerging from coma, mutism In 48 days: speech recovery After 12 months: consciousness state, critics decrease, right-sided hemiparesis	Severe disability	In 12 months: severe disability, right-sided hemiparesis

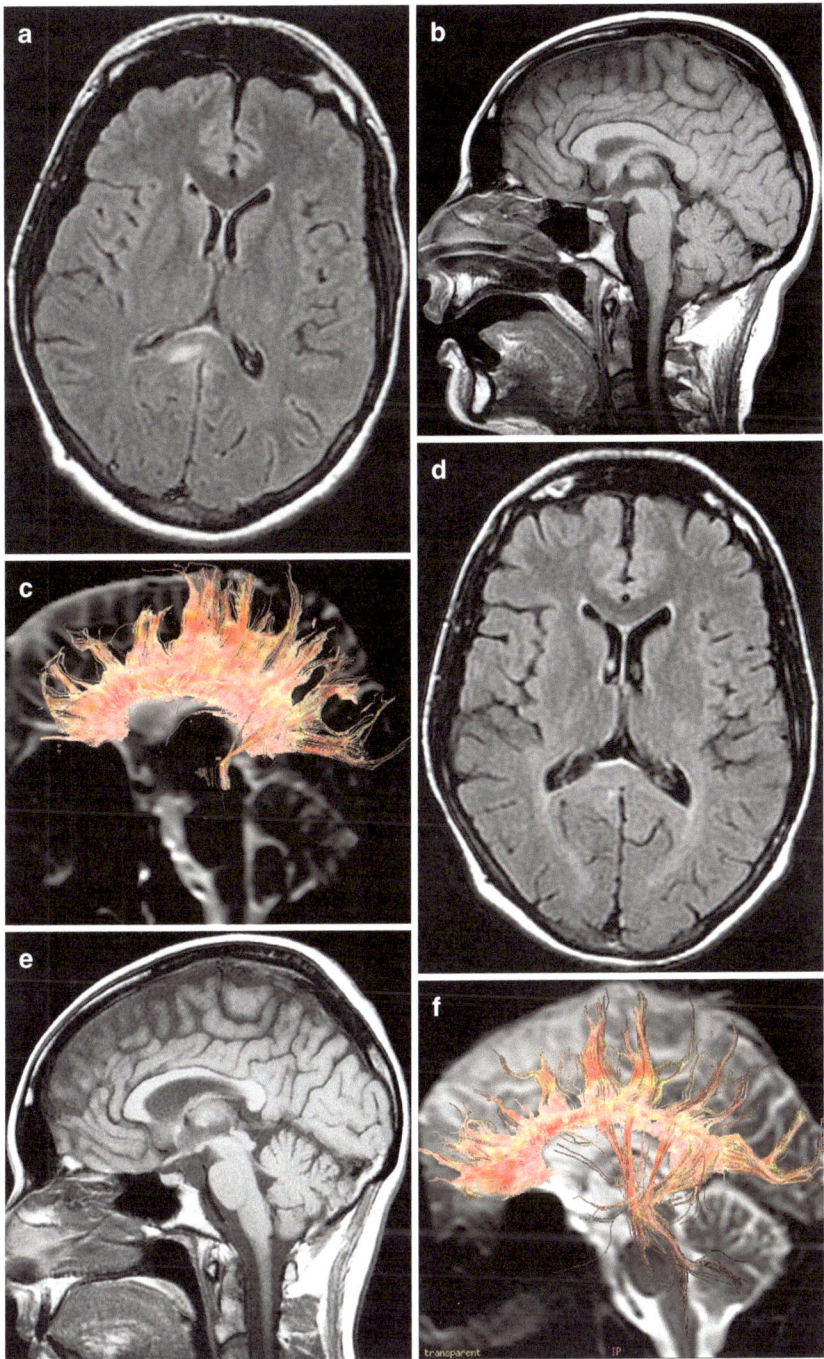

Fig. 4.4 Traffic accident. GCS, 5. Outcome, moderate disability. MRI, T2-FLAIR (**a**) shows a lesion in the splenium of the corpus callosum; T1 WI, (**b**) Tractography (**c**) in 15 days after injury does not reveal changes of the corpus callosum in a 3D reconstruction. MRI in 3 years after trauma: T2-FLAIR (**d**) no marked changes; T1 WI (**e**) atrophy of the corpus callosum; tractography (**f**) partial reduction in ascending fibers and loss of some fibers of the corpus callosum

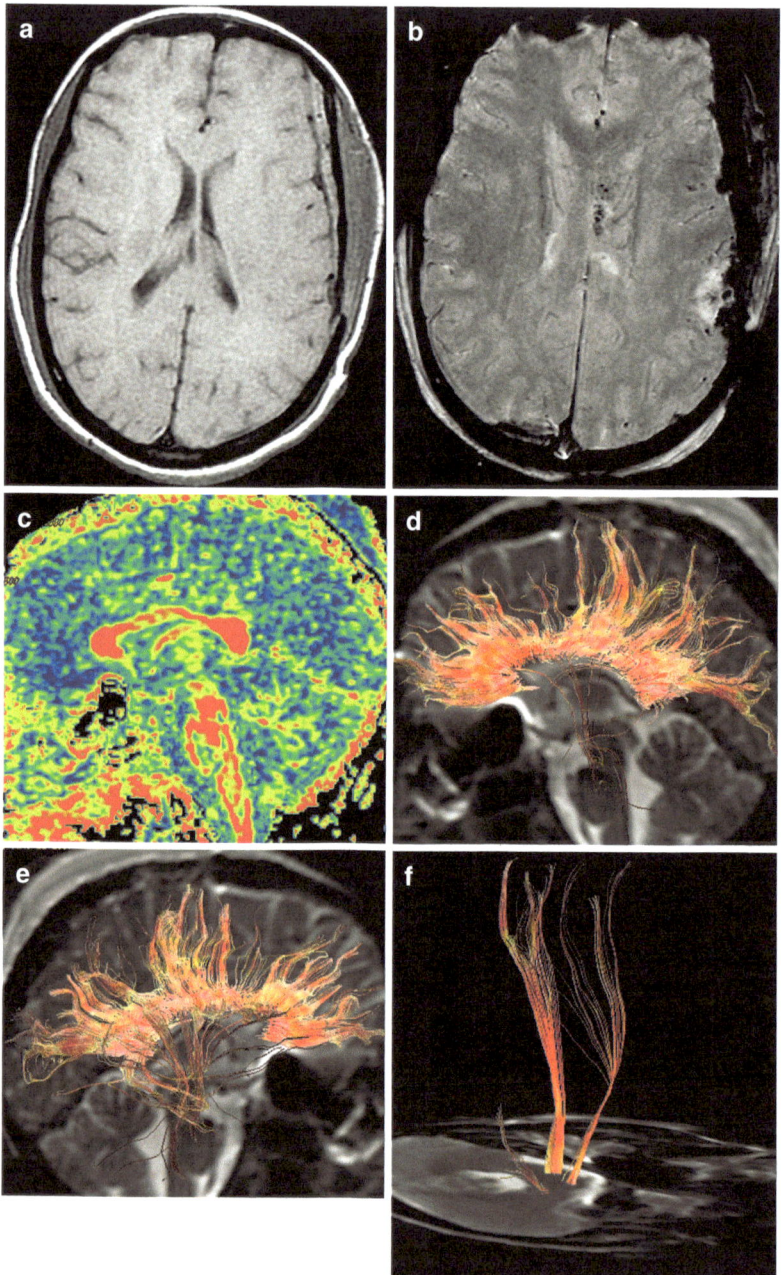

Fig. 4.5 Traffic accident. DAI. GCS, 6. Favorable outcome (moderate disability, mild left-sided hemiparesis, dysarthria). MRI study in 2 days after trauma, T1WI (**a**) subdural hematoma in the left frontoparietal region; SWAN modality (**b**) multiple microhemorrhages and edema in the corpus callosum and cingulum. Sagittal FA map (**c**) shows decrease of diffusion anisotropy in the middle part of the corpus callosum; tractography, no severe changes of the corpus callosum (**d, e**) slight asymmetry of the corticospinal tracts (R < S) (**f**) 32 days after injury, T1WI (**g**) reveals dilatation of subarachnoid spaces and ventricles; microhemorrhages in the corpus callosum and cingulum are preserved (SWAN, **h**); FA map (**i**) shows slight decrease of the corpus callosum in a midsagittal view. Tractography revealed reduction and shortening of fibers in the middle and posterior aspects of the corpus callosum, light asymmetry of CST is preserved (**j–l**)

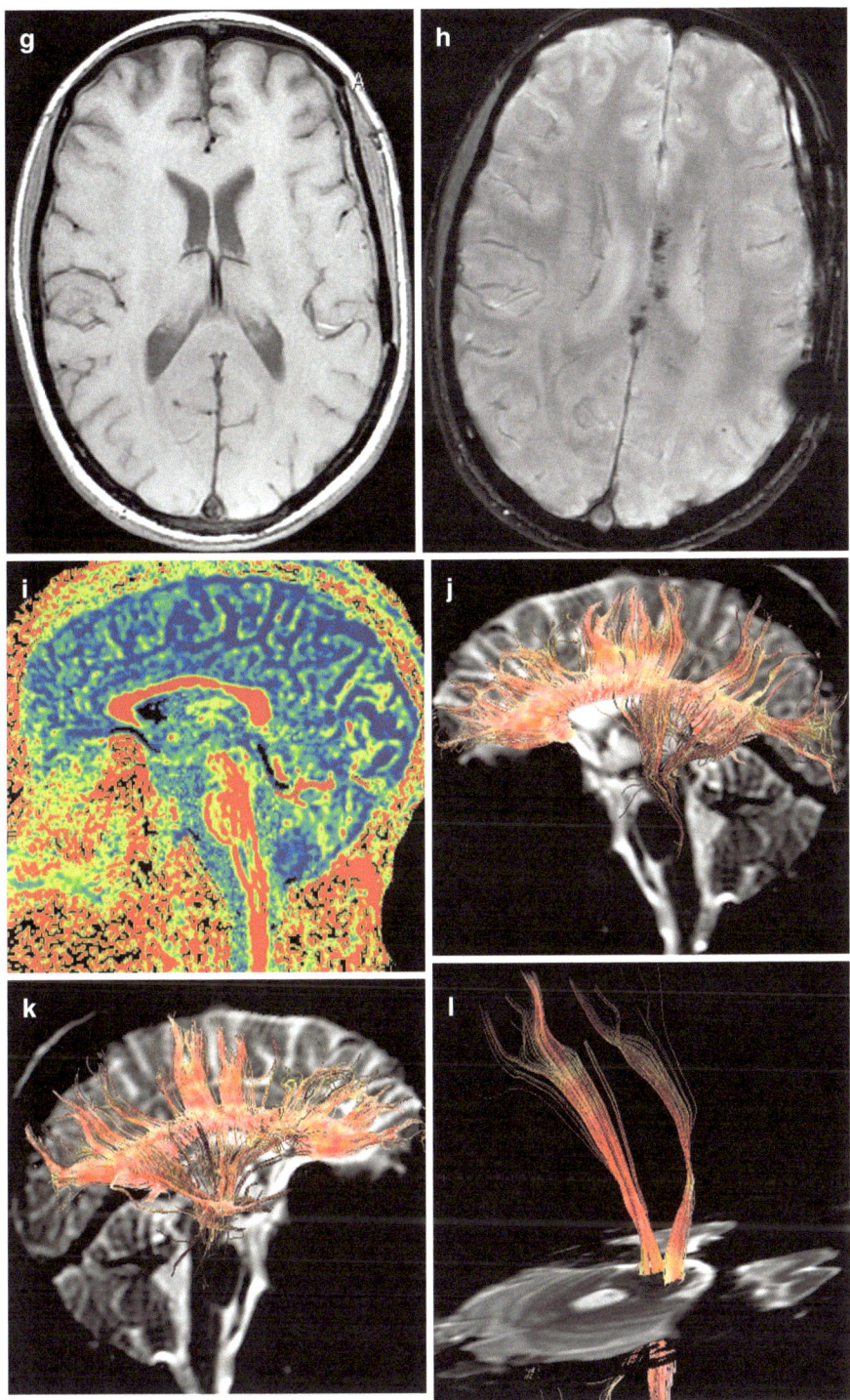

Fig. 4.5 (continued)

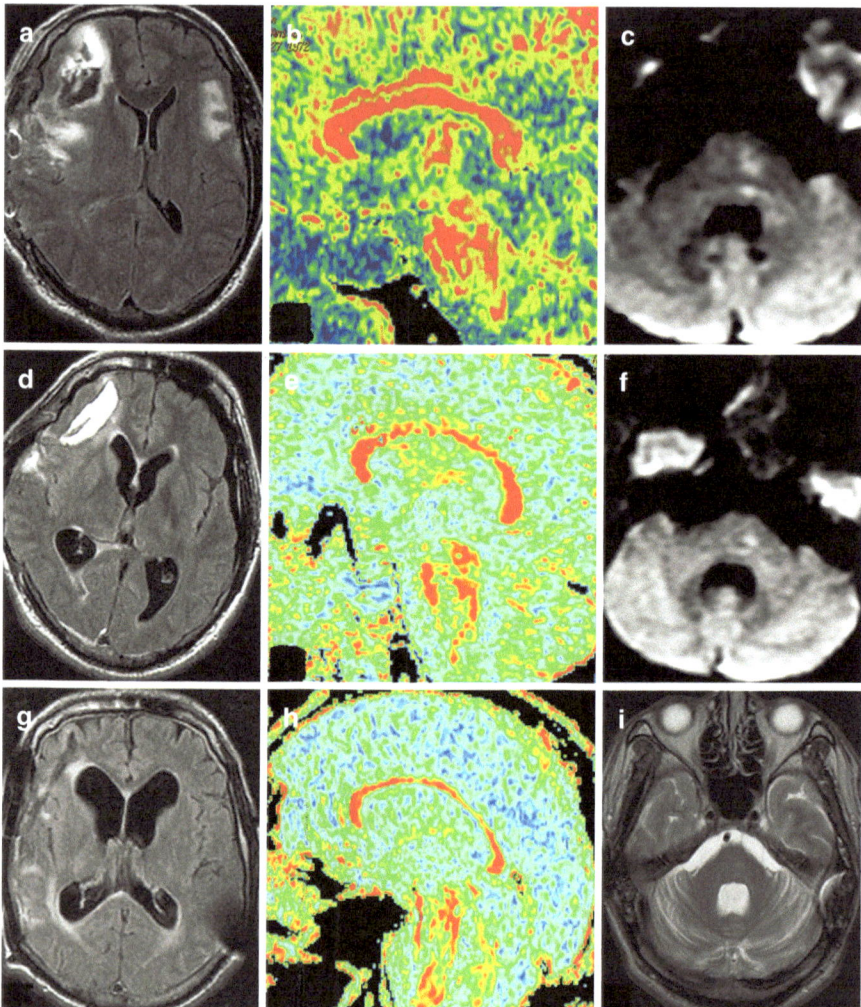

Fig. 4.6 Traffic accident. GCS, 5. DAI. Unfavorable outcome (vegetative state, minimally conscious state, tetraparesis). MRI: first examination in 5 days after trauma in T2-FLAIR (**a**); DWI (**c**) modalities show damages at the levels of the pons, corpus callosum, frontal lobes; on FA map (**b**), changes in the splenium of the corpus callosum. Second examination in 22 days, areas of MR signal change at the level of the pons are remained (**f**, DWI), ventricles are moderately enlarged (**d**, T2-FLAIR), atrophy of the corpus callosum and fractional anisotropy decrease (**e**, FA map). Third examination (in 19 months), further enlargement of ventricles and subarachnoid spaces, atrophic brain stem, and corpus callosum changes (**g**, T2-FLAIR; **h**, FA map; **i**, T2WI)

The other seven patients scanned in 3–20 weeks following injury (coma lasting 6–22 days) showed a significant thinning and loss of CC fibers with evidence of severe atrophy (Figs. 4.6 and 4.7). Three of these seven patients remained in the vegetative state and four in a state of severe disability with symptoms of serious mental and neurological disorders 3 months after the injury.

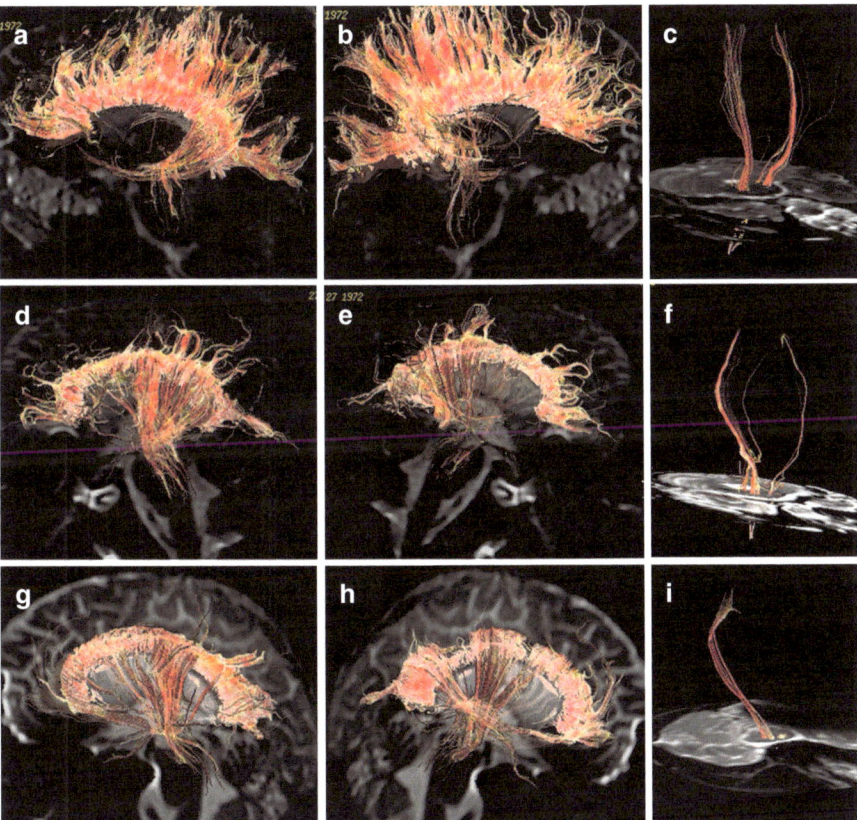

Fig. 4.7 Dynamics of MR tractography data in the same patient as in Fig. 4.6. First examination (in 5 days) reveals "defect" in the splenium of the corpus callosum, slight asymmetry of CST (**a**–**c**). Second examination (in 22 days) (**d**–**f**), shortening and decreasing of ascending fibers on the left. Third examination (in 19 months) (**g**–**i**), practically complete disappearance of ascending fibers of the corpus callosum; left corticospinal tract is not visible

Case Report (Figs. 4.6 and 4.7, Table 4.10, **patient 13**)

M., 34 y.o. Traffic accident. Diagnosis: diffuse axonal injury. Focal brain contusions in the right frontotemporoparietal region and left temporoparietal region. Subarachnoid hemorrhage.

Craniotomy and removal of the right parietal subdural hematoma, as well as left-sided decompressive craniectomy, were performed in a regional hospital. The patient was transferred to the Burdenko Neurosurgery Institute on the 2nd day after TBI. Neurological status: GCS, 5; signs of brain stem damage, mostly right-sided tetraparesis; spontaneous motor activity is absent; and left forearm flexion and right decerebrate reaction in response to nociceptive stimulation.

In 2 months after TBI, development of posttraumatic hydrocephalus, implanting of ventriculoperitoneal programmable shunt.

In 6 months after injury, bone defect plasty in the right parietal region.

In 8 months after TBI, the patient lies mostly with the eyes opened, strict gaze fixation when being addressed, performs simple right leg flexion-extension commands by repeated request, spontaneous active movements in lower extremities, upper extremities are adjacent to the body, and increased tonus.

Conclusion by a psychiatrist in 21 months after TBI, permanent depressed consciousness – emerging from vegetative to minimally conscious state (with gaze fixation and eye tracking, episodically obeying some commands and showing emotional reactions). Posttraumatic epilepsy and tetraparesis, more severe in the right arm.

GOS: vegetative state - minimally conscious state.

One of these seven patients was in the vegetative state and died within 7 months; five remained severely neurologically disabled (evident mental and neurological deficit). One patient in a state of severe neurological disability including hemiparesis recovered to a moderate degree of cognitive, emotional, and personality disorders in 1 year (Table 4.10, patients 10–14, 20–21, Fig. 4.8).

Figures 4.9 and 4.10 show dynamic MRI of a 39-year-old patient with diffuse and focal brain damage. He was in coma (GCS of 6) for 14 days and died after 7 months of being in a persistent vegetative state. As is seen from the figures, the first study (13 days post-injury) revealed a contusion of the right frontal lobe, damage of the corpus callosum with petechial hemorrhages (seen on T2*GRE), and bilateral subacute subdural hematomas. The follow-up study in 55 days after TBI (during vegetative state) revealed general brain atrophy, bilateral hygromas, and increasing degeneration of CC.

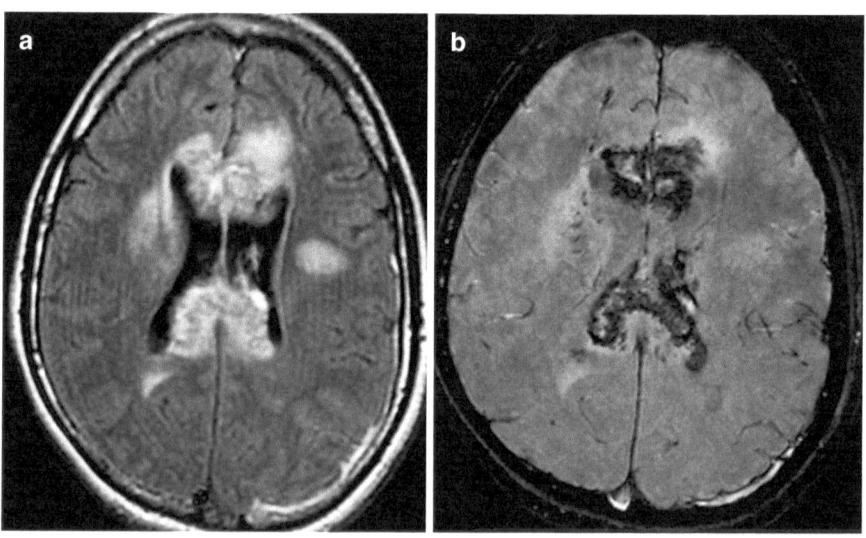

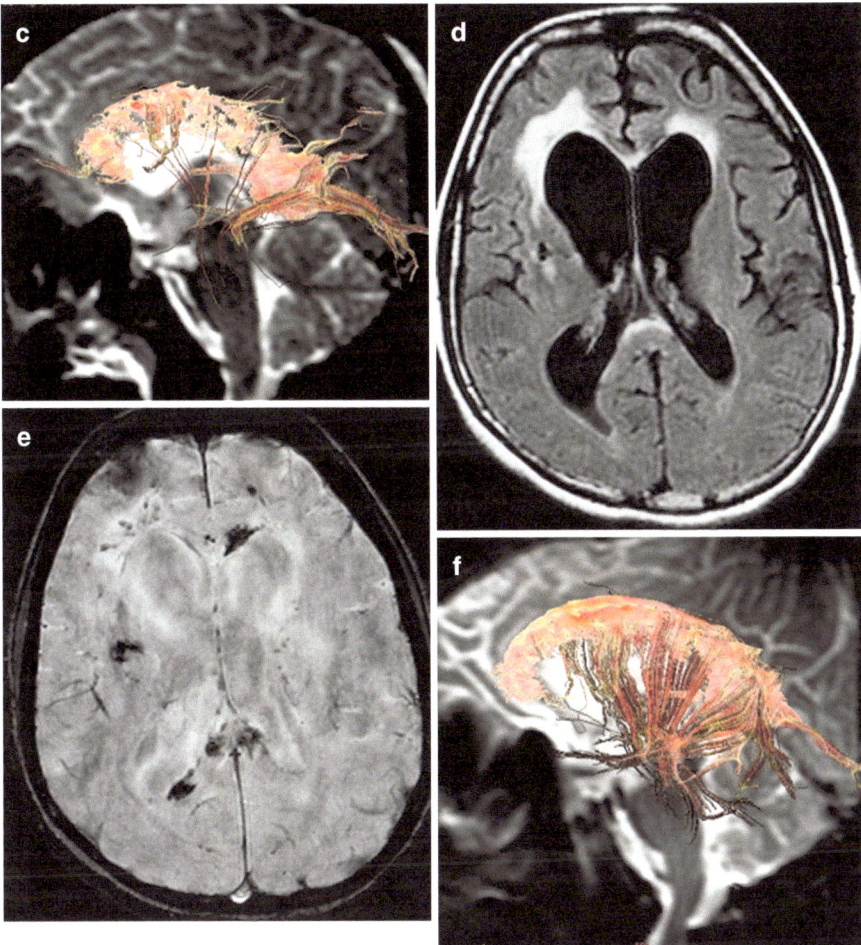

Fig. 4.8   (continued)

Fig. 4.8   Traffic accident. DAI. GCS, 4. MRI in 12 days after injury (T2-FLAIR, **a**; SWAN, **b**) demonstrates extensive areas of hemorrhagic damages of the corpus callosum, thinned ascending fibers of the corpus callosum in tractography (**c**). MRI study in 3 months (T2-FLAIR, **d**; SWAN, **e**), besides ventricular enlargement and areas of hemosiderin in the corpus callosum region, absence of ascending fibers of the CC in tractography is detected (**f**). Outcome in 3 months, severe disability; in 1 year, moderate cognitive, emotional, and personality disorders, left-sided hemiparesis

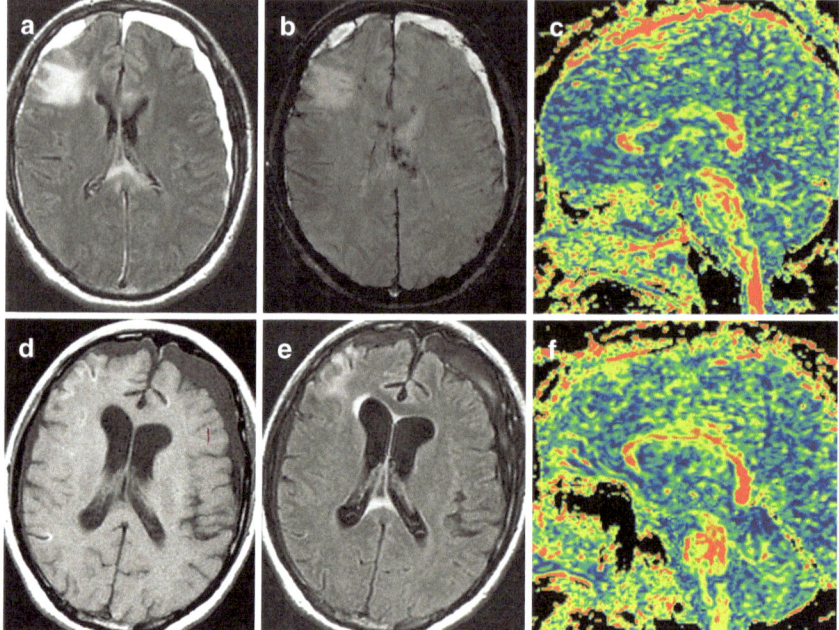

Fig. 4.9 Traffic accident. DAI. GCS, 6. GOS in 6 months, vegetative state, death in 7 months after injury. First MRI study (in 13 days after trauma): T2-FLAIR (**a**) and 3D GRE (**b**) reveal CC damages with microhemorrhages, focal contusion in the right frontal lobe, small subdural hematomas; FA map at midsagittal level (**c**) shows diffuse decrease of anisotropy in the corpus callosum. The second MRI study (in 55 days) visualizes enlargement of ventricles; areas of MR signal change are remained in the hemispheric structures and the corpus callosum, bilateral hygromas (T1WI, **d**; T2-FLAIR, **e**); on the FA map (**f**), diffuse atrophy of the corpus callosum, fractional anisotropy reduction

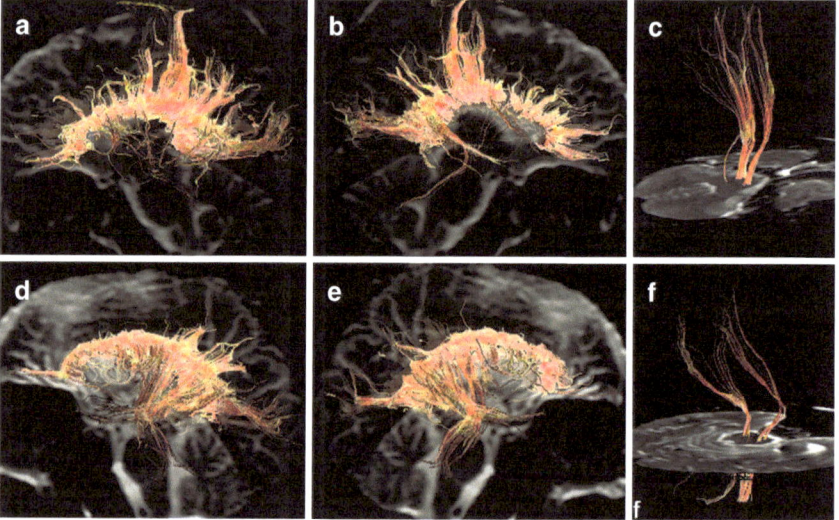

Fig. 4.10 Dynamic MR tractography in the same patient (see Fig. 4.9). The first MRI study in 13 days after trauma (**a–c**) reveals diffuse reduction of CC fibers (more in the anterior aspect and splenium region), slight asymmetry of CSTs (R<L). MRI study in 55 days (**d–f**) demonstrates a diffuse reduction and disappearance of the majority of CC fibers, "baldness of corpus callosum"

Case Report (Figs. 4.9 and 4.10, Table 4.10, **patient 14**)

M., 39 y.o. Traffic accident. Diagnosis: diffuse axonal injury, focal brain contusion in the right frontotemporal region, bilateral subdural hematomas in the right frontal and left frontotemporal regions, intraventricular and subarachnoid hemorrhage, and fractures of the anterior wall of the maxillary sinus, right zygomatic bone, and right clavicle.

On admission, GCS, 6; the patient reveals spontaneous motor activity with flexion of extremities and weak mimic reaction. Pupils are narrow; their reaction to light is preserved.

By the 10th day after TBI, patient's state is stabilized, emerged from coma into vegetative state, spontaneous movements in extremities are not marked, and brain stem dysfunction signs are absent. Eye opening in response to nociceptive stimuli, D=S, and pupils' response to light is normal. Patient does not respond to the addressed speech.

On the 22nd day after TBI, deterioration of patient's state with development of pneumonia and septic shock.

In 3.5 months after TBI, minimally conscious state and multiple organ dysfunction.

In 7 months after TBI, death caused by multiple organ dysfunction.

Morphological changes in CC were accompanied by a significant (in comparison with the control group) reduction in FA rates in the genu and the splenium ($p < 0.001$) and CST bilaterally (Table 4.11).

Table 4.11 Dynamics of averaged FA values in different brain structures in a 39-year-old patient, outcome: (death)

ROI		FA value ± SD (days after injury)		Differences between FA values in 13 and 55 days after injury	Differences (p) between FA values in patients and in control subjects	
		13	55	p	13	55
Genu of CC	R	0.496±0.076	0.55±0.159	0.075	0.001↓	0.001↓
	L	0.494±0.077	0.455±0.089	0.042↓	0.001↓	0.001↓
Splenium of CC	R	0.512±0.051	0.554±0.098	0.028↑	0.001↓	0.001↓
	L	0.51±0.1	0.521±0.092	0.597	0.001↓	0.001↓
PLIC	R	0.64±0.087	0.556±0.131	0.002↓	0.026↓	0.001↓
	L	0.595±0.12	0.52±0.128	0.008↓	0.007↓	0.001↓
Midbrain	R	0.5±0.11	0.499±0.074	0.973	0.001↓	0.001↓
	L	0.43±0.078	0.378±0.088	0.049↓	0.001↓	0.001↓
Pons	R	0.471±0.06	0.517±0.069	0.043↑	0.001↓	0.229
	L	0.424±0.11	0.406±0.068	0.649	0.001↓	0.001↓

ROI region of interest, *PLIC* posterior limb of the internal capsule, *CC* corpus callosum, *SD* standard deviation, *R* right, *L* left

The CSTs were bilaterally symmetrical in only 3 of 22 patients, both in the first and follow-up studies. Two of them had no signs of pyramidal tract damage and one patient had mild transient hemiparesis. No brain stem damage was detected on MRI scans (T1, T2, T2-FLAIR, DWI) in these 3 patients.

MRI demonstrated brain stem injury and asymmetry or bilateral reduction in the "density" of corticospinal tracts on tractography in 18 patients. All these patients had signs of pyramidal tract damage: hemi- and tetraparesis (Fig. 4.11).

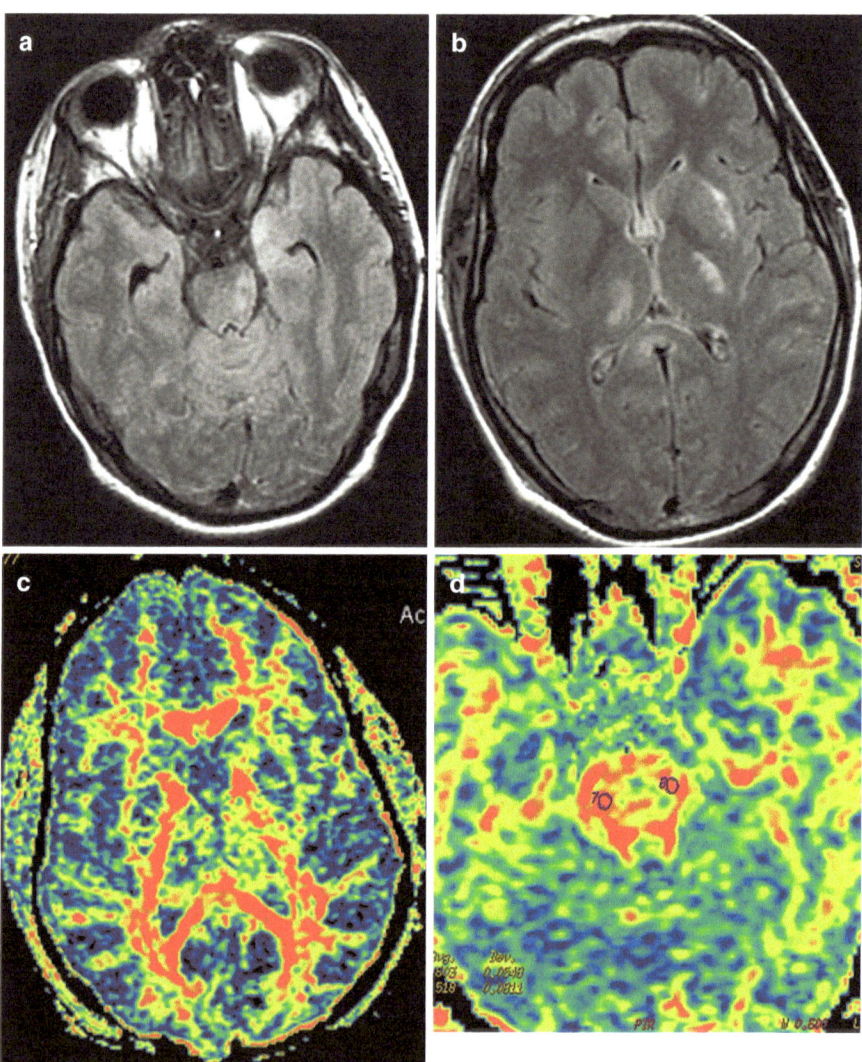

Fig. 4.11 DAI. GCS, 4. MRI study in 3 days after injury (T2-FLAIR, **a, b**; FA maps, **c, d**) shows lesions in the left cerebral peduncle, subcortical formations, corpus callosum; 3D reconstruction (**e**) reveals only slight asymmetry of CSTs. In 2 months after trauma, T2-FLAIR (**f**), atrophic hemispheric changes; FA map (**g**), marked decrease of fractional anisotropy parameters in the left cerebral peduncle area; tractography (**h**), left corticospinal tract atrophy. Outcome, severe disability, left-sided severe hemiparesis

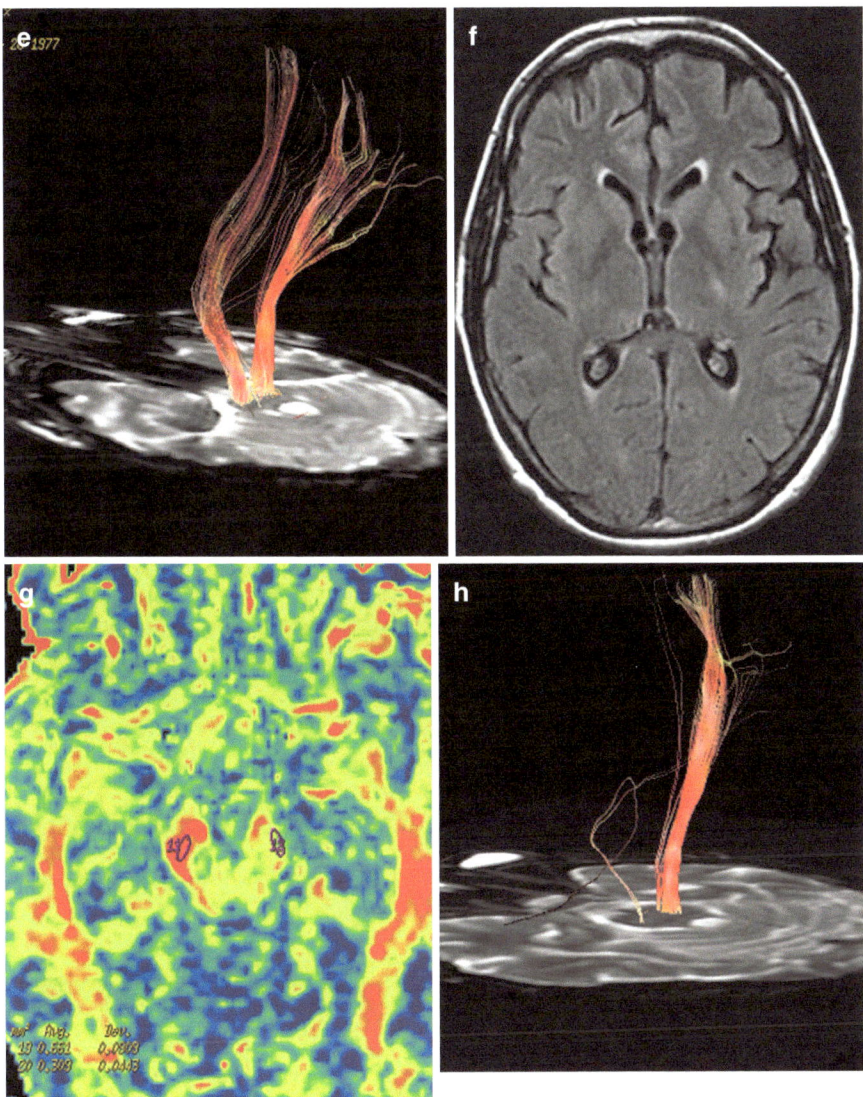

Fig. 4.11   (continued)

Case Report (Fig. 4.11)

F., 29 y.o. Traffic accident. Diagnosis: diffuse axonal injury.

On admission to the institute, GCS, 4; left extremity extension without localization in response to nociceptive stimuli; right-sided hemiparesis; pupils D = S; pupils' reaction to light and reflector vertical gaze are decreased; cough reflex is intact; and intracranial pressure, 15–18 mmHg.

By CT examination, diffuse brain edema, pathological density areas are not detected, and midline is not shifted. By perfusion CT, rCBF values are normal, without interhemispheric difference.

In 7 days after TBI, eye opening and more distinct arm flexion in response to nociceptive stimulation are marked.

In 14 days after TBI, the patient lies with opened eyes, blink reflex is weak, gaze is downward, pupils are equal, doesn't obey commands, corneal reflexes are depressed, and pupils' reaction to light is intact.

In 2 months after TBI, patient is able to obey commands, recognize members of the family, and left-sided spastic hemiparesis still remains.

GOS in 5 months: severe disability, right-sided hemiparesis with coordination and gait disorders, and clear consciousness with emotion and personality disturbances.

One patient, who was in coma for 20 days and underwent the first MRI study 8 days following trauma, had foci of increased signal in T2-FLAIR at the midbrain level, while tractography showed symmetry of CSTs. However, fractional anisotropy parameters at this level were lower on the right side. The patient had left-sided hemiparesis after emerging from coma. The second MRI study (29 days post-injury) revealed asymmetry of corticospinal tracts (Fig. 4.12).

Primary examinations of patients in 2–3 weeks after TBI demonstrated marked changes in the corpus callosum and corticospinal tracts (Fig. 4.13).

It should be emphasized that in all the analyzed patients, both the first and the second study showed decreased fractional anisotropy rates at different levels of CST on one or both sides.

A 23-year-old patient with severe DAI was scanned at 10, 37, and 77 days after trauma (Figs. 4.14 and 4.15, Table 4.12).

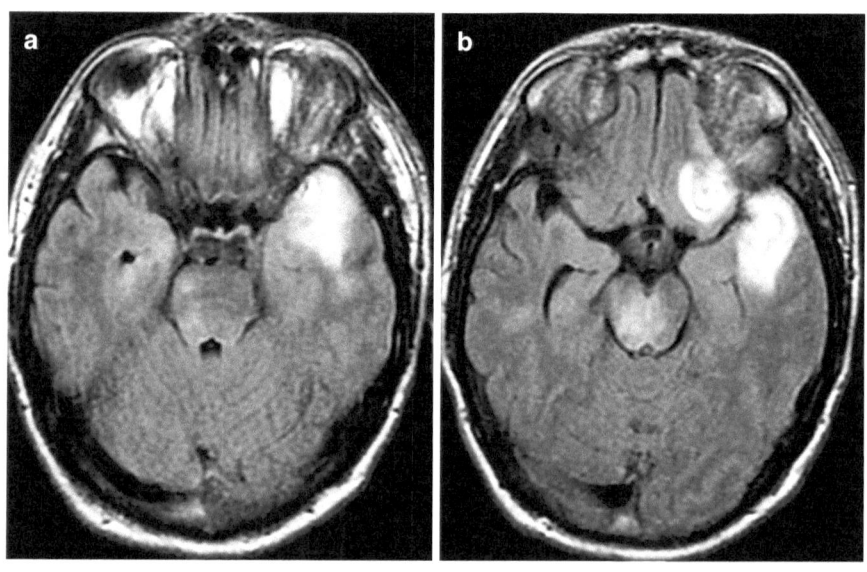

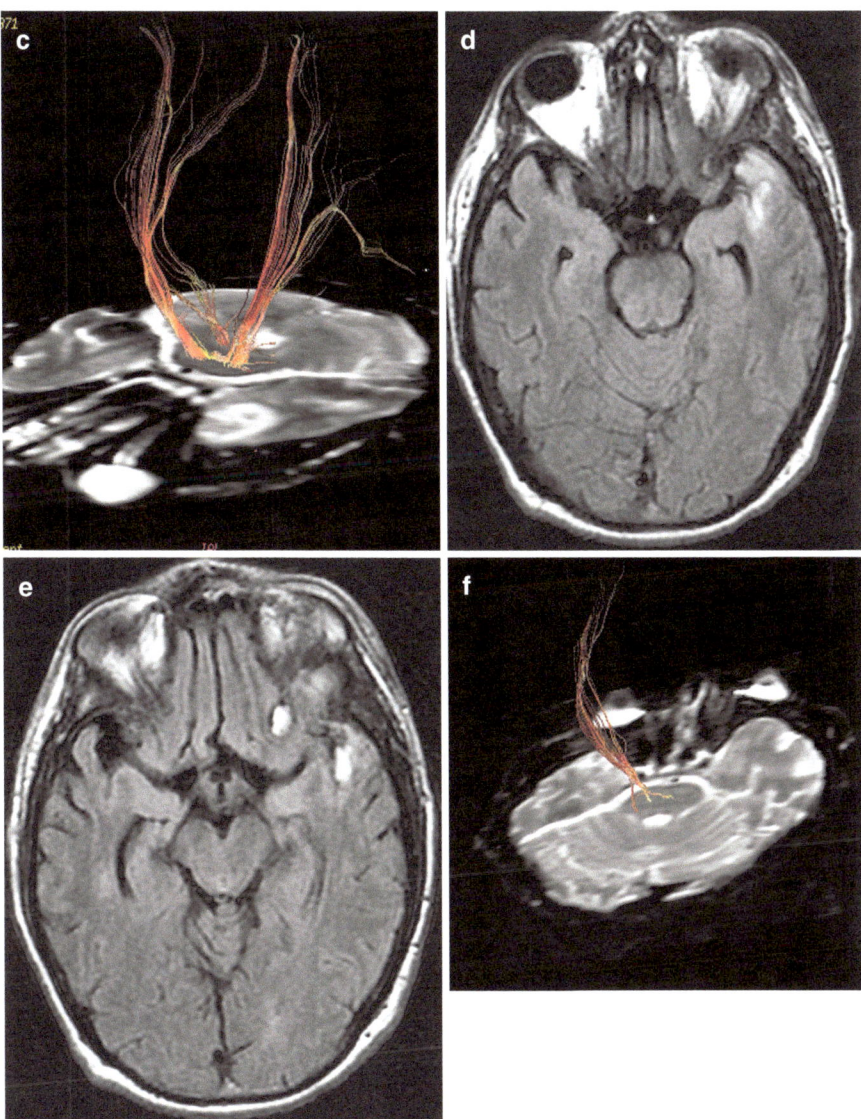

Fig. 4.12   (continued)

Fig. 4.12   DAI and focal brain contusions. GCS, 4. MRI in 8 days after injury: T2-FLAIR (**a**, **b**), damage zones in the right and middle parts of the midbrain, focal contusions in the left frontotemporal region; tractography (c); MRI study in 29 days after trauma, T2-FLAIR (**d**, **e**), moderate atrophic changes of the brain with basal cistern dilatation; tractography (**f**), disappearance of the right corticospinal tract

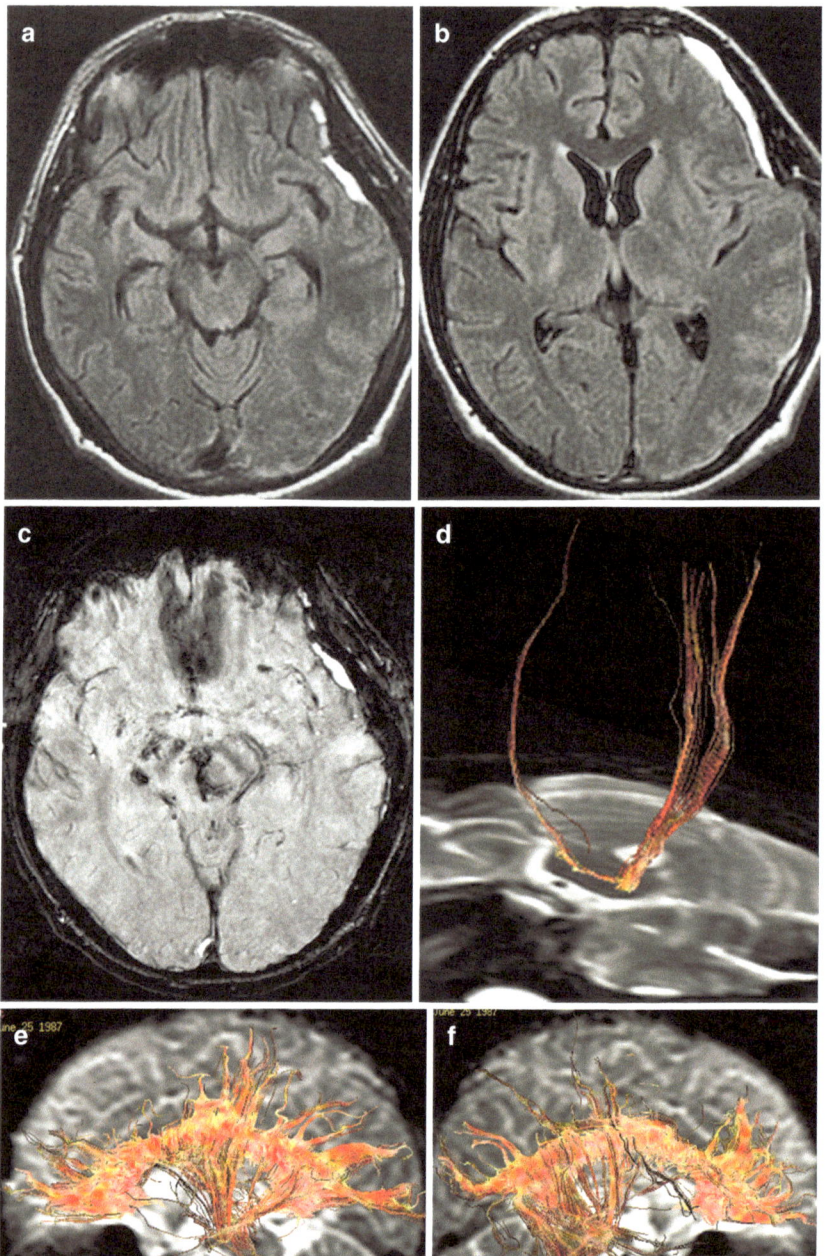

Fig. 4.13 Traffic accident. DAI, subdural hematoma in the left frontotemporal region. GCS, 5; coma duration 14 days. Outcome, severe disability, tetraparesis. MRI study in 18 days after trauma and emerging from coma (T2-FLAIR (**a**, **b**), SWAN (**c**)) shows subdural hematoma in the left frontotemporal region, hemorrhagic lesions in the midbrain; tractography (**d**–**f**), bilateral thinning of corticospinal tracts (more on the right), partial disappearance of ascending fibers of the corpus callosum (more on the right); MRI in 4 months after trauma (T2-FLAIR, **g**, **h**; SWAN, **i**) reveals atrophic brain changes, areas of hemosiderin deposition in the midbrain, subcortical formations (more on the right); in 3D reconstructions (**j**–**l**), unfavorable dynamics in the form of increased CST asymmetry, decreased volume of the corpus callosum fibers

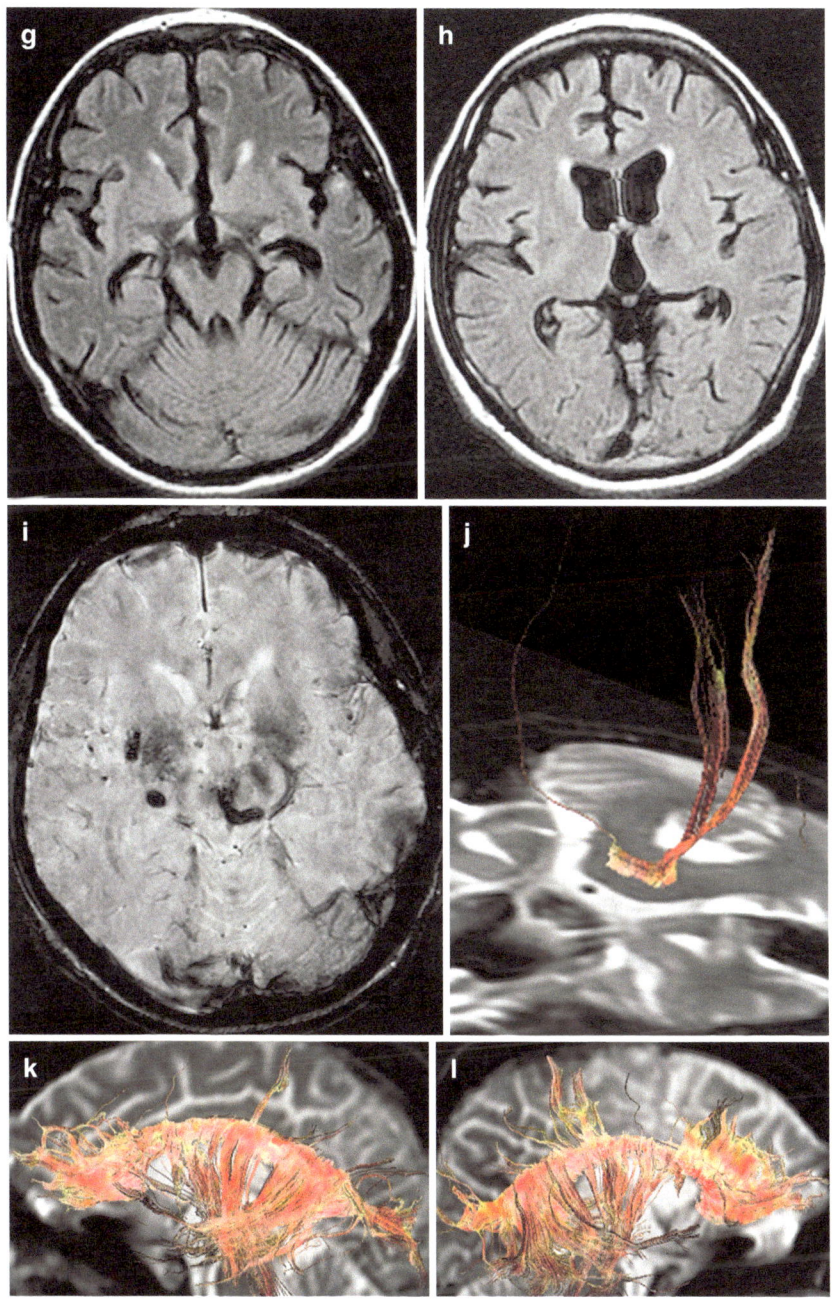

Fig. 4.13 (continued)

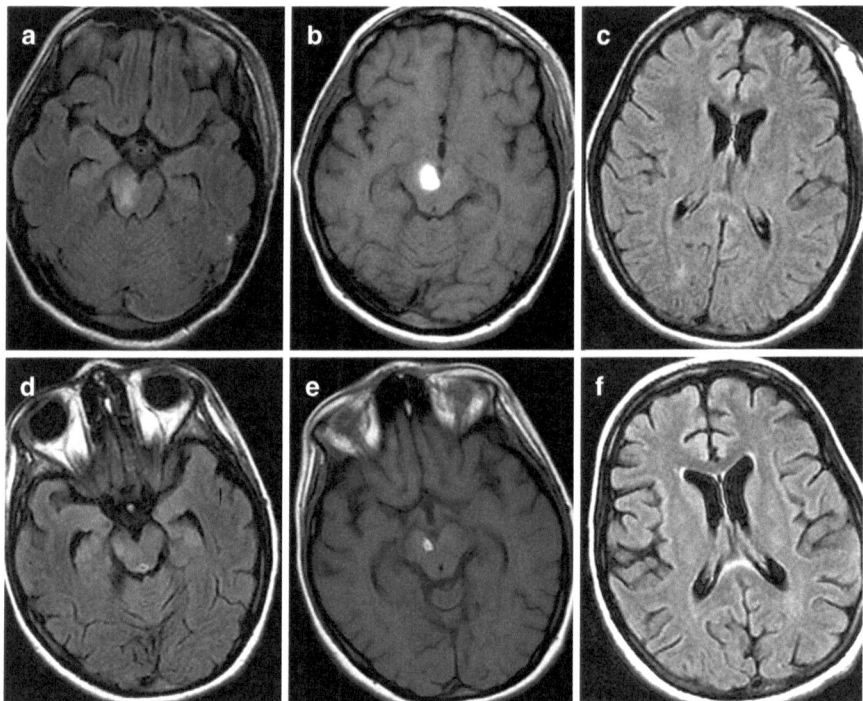

Fig. 4.14 F., 23 y.o. patient with DAI (after traffic accident) and unfavorable outcome (severe disability, severe left-sided hemiparesis). First MRI in 10 days reveals hemorrhagic areas in the right cerebral peduncle and medial region of the right thalamus, MR signal changes in the left part of the splenium of the corpus callosum (**a, c**, T2-FLAIR; **b**, T1WI). The second study in 37 days detects moderate diffuse brain atrophy, decreased size of hemorrhagic focus in the right cerebral peduncle (**d, f**, T2-FLAIR; **e**, T1 WI). In the third study (in 77 days), conventional MRI data did n't differ from those of the second MRI study

Case Report (Figs. 4.14 and 4.15, Table 4.10, **patient 5**)

F., 23 y.o. Traffic accident. Diagnosis: diffuse axonal injury with hemorrhagic lesions in the right cerebral peduncle and right part of the pons.

On admission, GCS, 5; gaze is fixed; anisocoria D>S; pupils are sluggishly reactive to light; corneal reflexes are depressed (mostly on the left side); and upgaze palsy.

CT study: diffuse brain edema with basal cistern compression and hemorrhagic lesion in the cerebral peduncle on the right.

Length of coma: 9 days.

Data of dynamic MRI studies in Figs. 4.14 and 4.15.

By the end of the 1st month, the patient comprehends the addressed speech, severe dysarthria is revealed, and severe left-sided hemiparesis is preserved.

After 6 months, clear consciousness; however, dysarthria, anisocoria, and severe left-sided hemiparesis are retained.

GOS in 6 months: severe disability and left-sided hemiparesis.

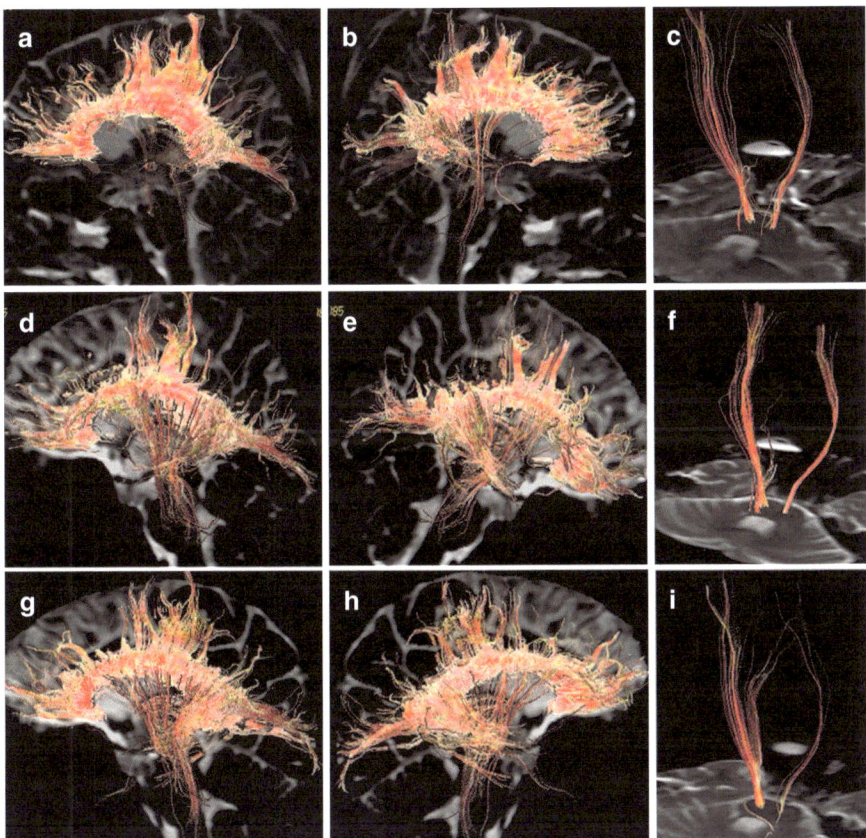

Fig. 4.15 F., 23 y.o. patient with DAI (after traffic accident) and unfavorable outcome (severe disability, severe left-sided hemiparesis); see Fig. 4.14. Dynamics of MR tractography data. MRI study in 10 days after injury (**a–c**) reveals partially shortening and disappearance of some fibers, mainly in the posterior part of the corpus callosum, slight asymmetry of CSTs. MRI studies in 37 (**d–f**) and 77 days (**g–i**) demonstrate unfavorable dynamics in the form of corpus callosum atrophy progression, more obvious asymmetry of CSTs – thinning of fibers on the right

The first examination (Figs. 4.14 and 4.15) revealed foci of damage in the splenium of CC and in the right side of the midbrain with a decreased number of corticospinal tract fibers on the right. This asymmetry became more obvious by the second and especially by the third study, 37 and 77 days after injury, respectively.

As is seen from Table 4.12, in the first study FA was significantly reduced in the genu and splenium of the CC compared to the healthy volunteers. A significantly reduced FA was observed along the CST at the level of the midbrain and PLIC on the right, as well as at the level of the pons bilaterally. The second study, conducted 37 days following the injury, revealed that FA values in the splenium and genu of the CC were significantly increased. This trend continued for 77 days post-injury. On the 9th day after injury, this patient displayed signs of emergence from coma as well as subsequent restoration of a verbal contact, but had a profound left-sided spastic hemiparesis. As is clear from Table 4.12, average values of FA on the right

Table 4.12 Dynamics of averaged FA values in different brain structures in a 23-year-old patient, outcome: severe disability

ROI		FA values ± SD (days after injury)			Differences (p) between FA values in patients and in control subjects		
		10	37	77	10	37	77
Genu of CC	R	0.731±0.01	0.758±0.11	0.745±0.1	0.013↓	0.623	0.875
	L	0.644±0.11*	0.725±0.11	0.728±0.06**	0.001↓	0.256	0.128
Splenium of CC	R	0.706±0.08*	0.763±0.11	0.727±0.05	0.001↓	0.183	0.001↓
	L	0.695±0.09*	0.733±0.06***	0.778±0.08**	0.001↓	0.001↓	0.570
PLIC	R	0.535±0.14*	0.675±0.07	0.652±0.07**	0.001↓	0.008↓	0.001↓
	L	0.681±0.14	0.692±0.07	0.695±0.055	0.272	0.266	0.31
Midbrain	R	0.551±0.19*	0.634±0.11	0.693±0.115**	0.001↓	0.0012↓	0.001↓
	L	0.745±0.01	0.724±0.09	0.765±0.104	0.001↑	0.386	0.008↑
Pons	R	0.438±0.09	0.406±0.12***	0.492±0.036	0.001↓	0.001↓	0.001↓
	L	0.515±0.06	0.469±0.08***	0.549±0.03	0.011↓	0.001↓	0.438

ROI region of interest, *PLIC* posterior limb of the internal capsule, *CC* corpus callosum, *SD* standard deviation, *R* right, *L* left
*$p < 0.05$, difference between averaged FA values in the 1st and 2nd MRI study; **$p < 0.05$, difference between averaged FA values in the 1st and 3rd MRI study; ***$p < 0.05$, difference between averaged FA values in the 2nd and 3rd MRI study

(along the CST) were significantly lower than on the left side. Furthermore, the values for both sides were significantly below normal during the last study; 16 months after injury the patient was still severely disabled with signs of severe left-sided spastic hemiparesis.

The progression of changes in the CC and CST in a 22-year-old patient who suffered from severe diffuse brain injury is shown on Figs. 4.16 and 4.17.

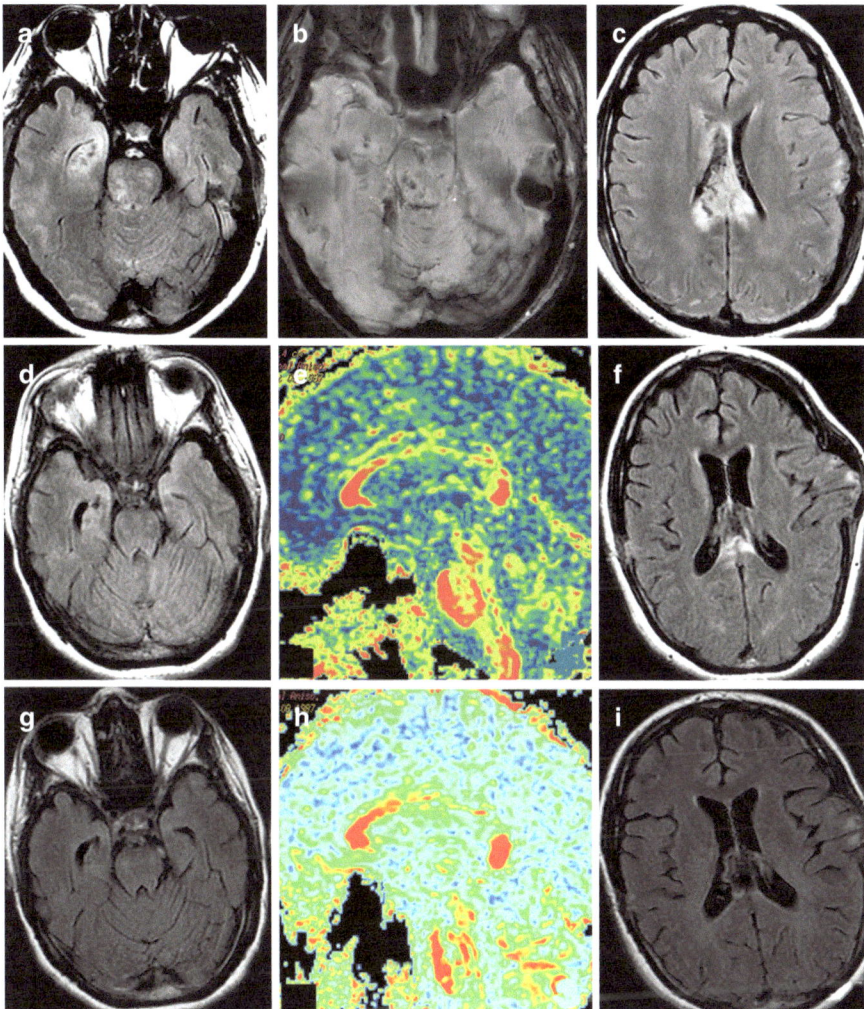

Fig. 4.16 F., 22 y.o. patient (after traffic accident) with DAI and unfavorable outcome (severe disability, tetraparesis). The first MRI study in 4 days after injury (in T2-FLAIR (**a, c**), SWAN (**b**) modalities) shows damaged areas at the level of the corpus callosum, midbrain, and pons. The second study in 33 days (T2-FLAIR (**d, f**), sagittal FA map (**e**)) and the third study in 4 months (T2-FLAIR, **g, i**; FA map, **h**) visualize hemispheric, brain stem, and corpus callosum atrophic changes

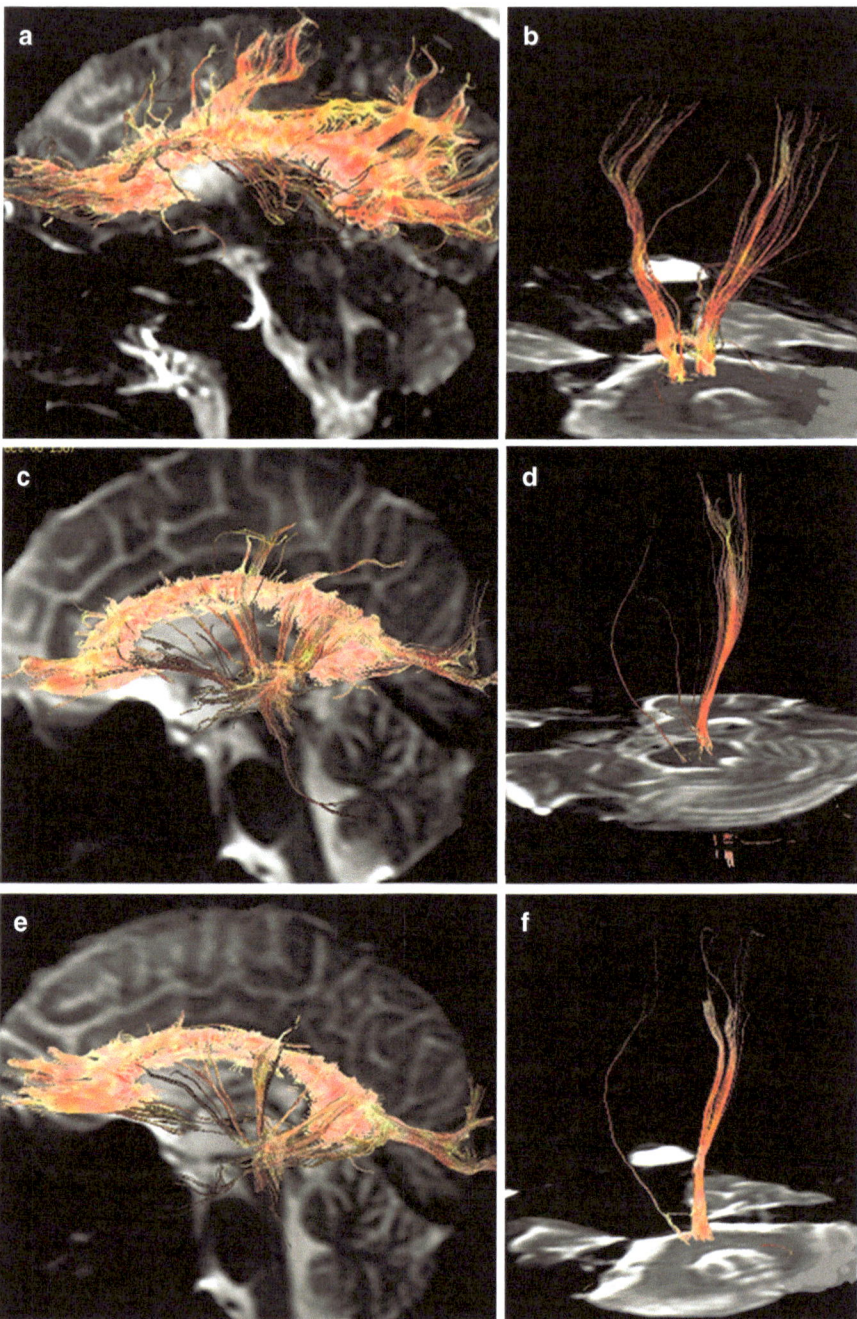

Fig. 4.17 Dynamics of MR tractography data in the same patient (see Fig. 4.16). First study (4 days after injury, **a, b**) reveals partial disappearance of the anterior part of corpus callosum fibers, symmetrical corticospinal tracts. Second MR tractography – in 33 days (**c, d**) – visualizes only some of the ascending fibers of the middle part, genu and splenium of the corpus callosum, corticospinal tracts asymmetry, thinning on the left. The third study (in 4 months after trauma, **e, f**) shows only isolated fibers in the genu and splenium of the corpus callosum ("baldness of corpus callosum"), asymmetric thinning of corticospinal tracts

Case Report (Figs. 4.16 and 4.17, Table 4.10, **patient 10**)

F., 22 y.o. Diagnosis: severe combined closed head injury, diffuse axonal injury, subarachnoid hemorrhage, and closed left clavicle fracture.

On admission, GCS, 4; episodes of decerebrate rigidity, spontaneous or due to nociceptive stimulation. Anisocoria D > S, pupils' reaction to light and corneal reflexes are depressed, oculocephalic reflex is absent, and severe tetraparesis.

By CT scans on admission, diffuse brain edema.

Dynamic MRI data are shown in Figs. 4.16 and 4.17.

By day 17, the patient's state is assessed as emergence from coma into vegetative state (spontaneous eye opening without gaze fixation). Signs of upper brain stem damage are preserved; mostly right-sided tetraparesis is marked.

In 1.5 months after TBI, speech comprehension and obeying some commands. Spastic tetraparesis with extrapyramidal signs and right-sided ptosis are preserved.

In 4 months after TBI, incomplete entrance into clear consciousness state with primary verbal attempts.

After 1.5 years, further positive dynamics, regression of motor aphasia, right third nerve insufficiency, moderate coordination disturbances, and slight regression of tetraparesis were marked.

GOS: severe disability.

Foci of damage of the corpus callosum and bilateral damage of the pons and midbrain were detected 4 days after the injury. At the same time, the structures of the CST were not changed significantly; CC fibers were partially nonvisualized. A follow-up study has been conducted 33 days after trauma after having emerged from coma to a vegetative state which proceeded to a state of akinetic mutism with signs of spastic tetraparesis. At the same time, DTI revealed a significant decrease in the number of CC fibers and CST asymmetry. The patient remained in severe disability state: aphasia and spastic tetraparesis (more severe on the right) 4 months after the injury. MR tractography at this time revealed almost complete reduction of the ascending CC fibers and CST asymmetry. Diffuse brain atrophy, including the corpus callosum and brain stem, was observed during MRI dynamic study. A neurological exam 8 months later revealed persistent tetraparesis, ataxia, motor aphasia, and dysarthria.

Thus, the studies show that in cases of diffuse axonal injury, changes in the structure of conductive pathways (corpus callosum, corticospinal tracts) can be observed already by the first 3–17 days after the initial injury. Such changes are most clearly seen 3–4 weeks after injury or later in patients with further vegetative state or severe disability. Degeneration of the CC and CST in such patients was accompanied by signs of diffuse brain atrophy, including the brain stem. These structural changes did not reach such a degree of severity in patients with moderate disability or good recovery.

4.3   Discussion

As was shown in studies of healthy volunteers, average ADC and FA values did not significantly differ on the symmetrical levels of both the corticospinal tracts. Data collected from 1.5T MRI were consistent with data from studies performed on 3T MRI. At the same time, average FA values along the CST at the pons level in healthy volunteers were significantly lower compared to FA values in the cerebral peduncles and posterior limb of the internal capsule on both sides. These results confirm the morphological evidence that CST fiber density at PLIC and peduncle levels is significantly higher compared to the pons level where transverse fibers intersect (Kamada et al. 2007; Haines 2008). Thus, the diffusion anisotropy values reliably reflect the degree of integrity and unidirectionality of conductive fibers of the brain. This aspect should be considered in studies of cerebral pathology.

It has been recently shown that in contrast to the routine MRI, diffusion-tensor MRI is invaluable in visualizing DAI in vivo on a "microstructural" level (Arfanakis et al. 2002; Huisman et al. 2004; Inglese et al. 2005). According to Bazarian et al. (2007) and Kim et al. (2008), this method is considered to be more sensitive for detecting axonal pathology in TBI.

According to the results of our study, there were extensive changes in structures of the white matter tracts of the CC and CST in the first 2–17 days after severe DAI accompanied by development of coma and different degrees of disability. These data have proved the results of earlier neuromorphological studies of DAI (Romodanovsky 1990; Kasumova 1998). FA parameters obtained in the early period following injury have proved to be the most sensitive indicator of white matter pathway damage in DAI. These studies have revealed a significant reduction in FA values compared to the norm for the corpus callosum and the corticospinal tracts at different levels in all the examined patients with severe DAI. Similar results were obtained by Huisman et al. (2004) for the splenium of CC and PLIC in 20 patients with a varying severity of head injuries within the first 7 days after TBI.

For a more detailed analysis of these results, the entire group of patients with DAI was divided into three subgroups: (1) with no obvious signs of pyramidal insufficiency, (2) with one-sided hemiparesis of different severity, and (3) with presence of tetraparesis. It is obvious that the second and third subgroups were characterized by a more severe degree of disability assessed by GOS in 6 months after injury. A characteristic feature of the first subgroup of patients with the most favorable outcome of DAI was a significant decrease in FA rates in all studied structures. However, there was no clear asymmetry of parameters at similar levels of the CST. At the same time, the FA rates at the level of PLIC and cerebral peduncles on the contralateral side of hemiparesis were significantly lower in patients of the second subgroup with clear clinical signs of unilateral pyramidal symptoms than in the control group. In addition, FA parameters along the CSTs differed significantly on homo- and contralateral to hemiparesis side at the level of PLIC and cerebral peduncles. These data confirm the results of Huisman et al. (2004) according to which the FA is a more sensitive indicator of pathway damage compared to ADC in the early period of TBI.

Four patients with tetraparesis in severe disability or vegetative state revealed the lowest bilateral FA values for all levels of the corticospinal tracts and ADC values for the pons level.

All the abovementioned data indicate that FA is absolutely reliable in reflecting the degree of damage to the corticospinal tracts in brain injury, which causes pyramidal insufficiency. These results support the studies of other authors. However, those studies were performed for patients with mild trauma or patients with different degrees of TBI severity at later stages of trauma (Arfanakis et al. 2002; Inglese et al. 2005; Wilde et al. 2006; Benson et al. 2007). A significant correlation between DAI outcome and values of FA in the corpus callosum and along the corticospinal tracts obtained 10–17 days after injury indicates a high predictive value of the diffusion anisotropy. It can be assumed that primary damage of white matter pathways in structures of the corticospinal tracts and corpus callosum in DAI leads to axonal degeneration resulting in a considerable decrease of FA values in 2–3 weeks after injury. These results confirm the data of van der Knaap (2005) that the primary brain damage, such as severe DAI, is a trigger of degenerative changes in axons and myelin sheaths leading to their complete destruction or atrophy in 2–3 months after trauma.

The role of the corpus callosum as the main structure responsible for interhemispheric communication has not yet been fully studied. Thus, in a series of studies of patients with congenital agenesia of the corpus callosum verified by modern neuroimaging techniques, a relatively normal development of higher cortical functions was marked (Gott and Saul 1978; Gazzaniga et al. 1989; Fisher et al. 1992; Quigley et al. 2003). However, only special psychological studies revealed patients' difficulties in solving the tasks requiring integration of visual, auditory, and tactile information of one-sided stimuli. Children with dysgenesia of the corpus callosum exhibited delayed verbal function development (Griebel et al. 1995). There is an opinion that the anterior commissure may take part in an interhemispheric integration in patients with congenital agenesia of the corpus callosum (Fisher et al. 1992; Corballis and Finlay 2000).

Long-term studies of the "split brain" in patients who underwent callosotomy for severe forms of epilepsy made a fundamental contribution to determining the role of the corpus callosum in brain functioning (van Wagenen and Herren 1940; Akelatis 1944; Myers and Sperry 1958; Bogen and Vogel 1962; Sperry and Gazzaniga 1967, 1969; Gazzaniga 1982, 2000, 2005). It has been shown that the splitting of the corpus callosum blocks interhemispheric transmission of sensory, motor, gnostical, and other types of information. This allowed specifying interhemispheric differences and mechanisms of interhemispheric interaction.

Examinations of patients with a localized damage of the corpus callosum revealed that the posterior regions of the CC are involved primarily in transmission of sensory information (visual, auditory, somatosensory), while the anterior are involved in transmission of cognitive information (Gazzaniga and Freedman 1973, 1982, 2000; Reisse et al. 1989; Jhori et al. 2000; Buklina 2001, 2004; Fabri et al. 2001).

In our opinion, the diffuse axonal injury is a different model of a *multidimensional split brain* as a result of damage to commissural (interhemispheric), association (intrahemispheric), and projection (cortical-subcortical and corticospinal, etc.)

connections. Examinations of individuals with congenital agenesia of the corpus callosum and callosotomy help to suggest that damage of the corpus callosum with its global atrophy cannot be the main cause of unrestored consciousness in patients with severe DAI. In our series, in patients with MRI signs of damage and subsequent development of atrophy of the corpus callosum and brain stem, the emergence from unconscious state to a minimally conscious state was possible either through a transient vegetative state or long-term period of disintegrated consciousness with persistent disturbances of mental functions (orientation, memory, speech, etc.) (Table 4.10). However, our observations showed that MR tractography in patients with relatively fast and full mental recovery activity in a few weeks or months after DAI revealed that the structures of the corpus callosum remained either normal or were only partially degenerated in dynamics (Zakharova et al. 2010a, b; Zakharova 2013).

Unilateral or bilateral damage and subsequent degeneration of the corticospinal tracts as well as signs of brain stem damage were identified in 18 of 22 patients studied by DT-MRI in dynamics. Our data confirm other authors' findings (Yasokawa et al. 2007) that severe damage of the projection pathways is one of the most characteristic features of severe DAI. Moreover, the degree of primary damage of the projection, commissural, or association connections is determined in each specific case by predominant biomechanics of the linear, angular, and rotational effects. Further structural changes and functional outcome also depend on the severity of secondary mechanisms of injury (edema, ischemia, hypoxia, etc.). Our studies showed that damage of the corpus callosum and corticospinal tracts with further obvious development of atrophy in severe DAI cases was observed in patients with partial conscious, mental, and motor recovery (minimally conscious state or disintegrated consciousness, hemi- and tetraparesis) or in patients in a persistent vegetative state.

The data obtained suggest that duration of pathway degeneration in DAI should cover a period from several weeks to 8–12 months. Previously published results of morphological and MRI studies have also confirmed these findings (Blatter et al. 1997; Povlishock 2000; Meythaler et al. 2001; Naganawa et al. 2004; Tomaiuolo et al. 2004; Bigler et al. 2006; Schiff 2006; Ding et al. 2008; Sidaros et al. 2008).

The most intriguing question remains, whether it is possible to identify not only destruction and degeneration but also regeneration of pathways by modern neuroimaging techniques. Our clinical observations and data of other authors indicate that mental recovery in several months and even years after prolonged vegetative state or minimally conscious state is possible even after severe injury. Increased rates of fractional anisotropy in our dynamic studies of individual patients as well as several observations of other authors (Voss et al. 2006; Sidaros et al. 2008) do not exclude such a possibility.

Further studies using DT-MRI at different stages of TBI will help to determine quantitative and qualitative changes in white matter tracts of the brain as well as their clinical correlations, which will allow a deeper understanding of TBI pathogenesis.

References

Akelatis A (1944) A study of gnosis, praxis and language following section of the corpus callosum and anterior commissure. J Neurosurg 1:94–102

Arfanakis K, Haughton V, Carew J et al (2002) Diffusion tensor MR imaging in diffuse axonal injury. AJNR Am J Neuroradiol 23:794–802

Bazarian J, Zhong J, Blyth B et al (2007) Diffusion tensor imaging detects clinically important axonal damage after mild traumatic brain injury: a pilot study. J Neurotrauma 24:1447–1459

Benson R, Meda S, Vasudevan S et al (2007) Global white matter analysis of diffusion tensor images is predictive of injury severity in traumatic brain injury. J Neurotrauma 24:446–459

Bigler E, Ryser D, Gandhi P et al (2006) Day-of-injury computerized tomography, rehabilitation status, and development of cerebral atrophy in person with traumatic brain injury. Am J Phys Med Rehabil 85:793–806

Blatter D, Bigler E, Gale S et al (1997) MR-based brain and cerebrospinal fluid measurement after traumatic brain injury: correlation with neuropsychological outcome. AJNR Am J Neuroradiol 18:1–10

Bogen J, Vogel P (1962) Cerebral commissurotomy in man. Bull Los Angel Neurol Soc 27:169–172

Buklina S (2001) The phenomenon of unilateral spatial ignorance in patients with arteriovenous malformations of deep brain structures. Zh Neurol Psikhiatr im SSKorsakova 101:10–15

Buklina S (2004) Corpus callosum, interhemispheric interaction and brain right hemisphere function. Zh Neurol Psikhiatr im SSKorsakova 5:8–14

Corballis M, Finlay D (2000) Interhemispheric visual integration in three cases of familial callosal agenesis. Neuropsychology 14:60–70

Ding K, Marquez de la Plata C, Wang J et al (2008) Cerebral atrophy after traumatic white matter injury: correlation with acute neuroimaging and outcome. J Neurotrauma 25:1433–1440

Fabri M et al (2001) Posterior corpus callosum and interhemispheric transfer of somatosensory information: an fMRI and neuropsychological study of partially callosotomized patient. J Cogn Neurosci 13:1071–1079

Fisher M, Ryan S, Dobyns W (1992) Mechanisms of interhemispheric transfer and patterns of cognitive function in acallosal patients of normal intelligence. Arch Neurol 49:271–277

Gazzaniga M (1982) Split brain research: a personal history. Cornell Univ Alumi Q 45:2–12

Gazzaniga M (2000) Cerebral specialization and interhemispheric communication: does the corpus callosum enable the human condition? Brain 123:1293–1326

Gazzaniga M (2005) Forty-five years of split-brain research and still going strong. Nat Rev Neurosci 6:653–659

Gazzaniga M, Freedman H (1973) Observations on visual processes after posterior callosal section. Neurology 23:1123–1130

Gazzaniga M, Kutas M, van Petten C, Fendrich R (1989) Human callosal function: MRI-verified neuropsychological functions. Neurology 39:942–946

Gott P, Saul R (1978) Agenesis of the corpus callosum: limits of functional compensation. Neurology 28:1272–1279

Griebel M, Williams J, Russel S et al (1995) Clinical and developmental findings in children with giant interhemispheric cysts and dysgenesis of the corpus callosum. Pediatr Neurol 13:119–124

Haines D (2008) Neuroanatomy. An atlas of structures, sections and systems (trans: Bobylova M). Logosphere, Moscow, p 116–137. English edition: Haines D (2004) Neuroanatomy. An atlas of structures, sections and systems. Lippincott Williams &Wilkins, Baltimore/Philadelphia

Huisman T, Schwamm L, Schaefer P et al (2004) Diffusion tensor imaging as potential biomarker of white matter injury in diffuse axonal injury. AJNR Am J Neuroradiol 25:370–376

Inglese M, Makani S, Johnson G et al (2005) Diffuse axonal injury in mild traumatic brain injury: a diffusion tensor imaging study. J Neurosurg 103:298–303

Jhori N, Kawamura M, Fukuzawa K et al (2000) Somesthetic disconnection syndromes in patients with callosal lesions. Eur Neurol 44:65–71

Kamada K, Sawamura Y, Takeuchi F (2007) Functional identification of the primary motor area by corticospinal tractography. In: Appuzo M (ed) Surgery of the human cerebrum. Lippincott Williams &Wilkins, Hagerstown, pp 166–176

Kasumova S (1998) Pathologic anatomy of traumatic brain injury. In: Konovalov A, Likhterman L, Potapov A (eds) Clinical guidelines on traumatic brain injury, vol 1, Antidor, Moscow, p 169–229

Kim J, Avants B, Patel S et al (2008) Structural consequences of diffuse traumatic brain injury: a large deformation tensor-based morphometry study. Neuroimage 39:1014–1026

Marshall L, Marshall S, Klauber M, Clark M (1991) A new classification of head injury based on computerized tomography. J Neurosurg 75:14–20

Meythaler J, Peduzzi J, Eleftherion E, Novack T (2001) Current concepts: diffuse axonal injury – associated traumatic brain injury. Arch Phys Med Rehabil 82:1461–1471

Myers R, Sperry R (1958) Interhemispheric communication through the corpus callosum: mnemonic carry-over between the hemispheres. Arch Neurol Psychiatry 80:298–303

Naganawa S, Sato C, Ishihra S et al (2004) Serial evaluation of diffusion tensor brain fiber tracking in a patient with severe diffuse axonal injury. AJNR Am J Neuroradiol 25:1553–1556

Potapov A, Kravchuk A, Zakharova N (2009) Head trauma. In: Kornienko V, Pronin I (eds) Diagnostic neuroradiology. Springer, Heidelberg, pp 807–919

Povlishock J (2000) Pathophysiology of neural injury: therapeutic opportunities and challenges. Clin Neurosurg 46:113–126

Quigley M, Cordes D, Turski P et al (2003) Role of the corpus callosum in functional connectivity. AJNR Am J Neuroradiol 24:208–212

Reisse G et al (1989) Interhemispheric transfer in patients with incomplete section of the corpus callosum. Anatomic verification with magnetic resonance imaging. Arch Neurol 46:437–443

Romodanovsky P (1990) Forensic-medical diagnosis of diffuse axonal brain damage in head injury. Dissertation, Second Medical institute, Moscow

Schiff N (2006) Multimodal neuroimaging approaches to disorders of consciousness. J Head Trauma Rehabil 21:388–397

Sidaros A, Engberg A, Sidaros K et al (2008) Diffusion tensor imaging during recovery from severe traumatic brain injury and relation to clinical outcome: a longitudinal study. Brain 131:559–572

Sperry R, Gazzaniga M (1967) Language following surgical disconnection of the hemispheres. In: Darley F (ed) Brain mechanisms underlying speech and language. Grune and Stratton, New York, p 108–121

Sperry R, Gazzaniga M, Bogen J (1969) Interhemispheric relationships: the neocortical commissures; syndromes of hemisphere disconnection. In: Vinken PJ, Bruyn GW (eds) Handbook of clinical neurology. North Holland, Amsterdam

Tomaiuolo F, Carlesino G, Di Paola M et al (2004) Gross morphology and morphometric sequelae in the hippocampus, fornix and corpus callosum of patients with severe non-missile without macroscopically detectable lesion: a T1-weighted MRI study. J Neurol Neurosurg Psychiatry 75:1314–1322

van der Knaap M (2005) Wallerian degeneration and myelin loss secondary to neuronal and axonal degeneration. In: van der Knaap M (ed) Magnetic resonance of myelination and myelin disorders, 3rd edn. Springer, Heidelberg, pp 832–839

van Wagenen W, Herren R (1940) Surgical division of commissural pathways in the corpus callosum: relation to spread of an epileptic attack. Arch Neurol Psychiatry 44:740–759

Voss H, Ulug A, Dyke J et al (2006) Possible axonal regrowth in late recovery from the minimally conscious state. J Clin Invest 116(7):2005–2011

Wilde E, Chu Z, Bigler E et al (2006) Diffusion tensor imaging in the corpus callosum in children after moderate to severe traumatic brain injury. J Neurotrauma 23:1412–1426

Yasokawa Y, Shinoda J, Okumura A et al (2007) Correlation between diffusion- tensor resonance imaging and motor-evoked potential in chronic severe diffuse axonal injury. J Neurotrauma 241:163–173

Zakharova N (2013) Neuroimaging of structural and hemodynamic disturbances in severe traumatic brain injury (clinical CT – MRI studies). Dissertation, Burdenko neurosurgery institute, Moscow

Zakharova N, Potapov A, Kornienko V et al (2010a) Assessment of brain pathways in diffuse axonal injury using diffusion-tensor MRI. Zh Vopr Neurokhir im NNBurdenko 2:3–9

Zakharova N, Potapov A, Kornienko V et al (2010b) Dynamic assessment of corpus callosum and corticospinal tracts structure using diffusion-tensor MRI in diffuse axonal injury. Zh Vopr Neurokhir im NNBurdenko 3:3–9

Mapping of Cerebral Blood Flow in Focal and Diffuse Brain Injury

Contents

5.1 Clinical Material 107
5.2 Peculiarities of rCBF in Patients with Diffuse Axonal Injury 112
5.3 Peculiarities of rCBF in Patients with DAI Combined with Focal Brain Contusions 115
5.4 Peculiarities of rCBF in Patients with Focal Brain Contusions 117
5.5 Peculiarities of rCBF in the Contusion Areas... 119
5.6 Study of rCBF in Subcortical Formations (Basal Ganglia and Thalami) 119
5.7 Discussion 119
References... 122

5.1 Clinical Material

Clinical material included 40 patients with severe TBI, aged 16–54 years (average 31 ± 10.4), 29 males and 11 females. Brain trauma was caused by traffic accidents in 27 cases (67.5 %), assaults or fights in 10 (25 %) cases, and falls from one's own or great heights in 3 (7.5 %) cases. Twelve patients had DAI of I–III CT categories (Marshall et al. 1991); 15 patients had DAI combined with focal cortical-subcortical contusions, including 5 patients with subdural hematomas. CT in 13 patients (32.5 %) revealed prevailing features of focal contusion; in 6 of them it was combined with epidural or subdural hematomas. Twenty-six patients (65 %) had concomitant trauma.

The severity of brain injury according to Glasgow Coma Scale at admission ranged 4–8 (average 6 ± 1.5) (Teasdale and Jennett 1974). Thirteen of 40 (30 %) patients had a lucid interval before admission; 19 (47.5 %) of 40 patients underwent surgery for intracranial hematomas, impressed skull fractures, and basal CSF leakage; 10 (25 %) of 40 patients underwent decompressive craniectomy (uni- or bilateral) due to increased intracranial hypertension and inefficient conservative treatment.

Four healthy volunteers without history of neurological disease or significant head trauma were studied using the same CT perfusion parameters; age range was 21–36 (mean = 30) (Pronin et al. 2007).

Table 5.1 shows the main characteristics and statistical data on the analyzed group of patients, including TBI severity by GCS, coma duration, outcome by GOS, CT findings, and ICP and CPP monitoring data.

GCS has proved to be an adequate general indicator of TBI severity for the whole group of patients due to its strong correlation with outcome by GOS ($R = 0.73$, $p < 0.01$). A significant correlation ($p < 0.05$) has been found between GCS, on the one hand, and presence or absence of the lucid interval ($R = 0.31$), degree of basal cistern compression ($R = -0.65$), presence or absence of the intraventricular hemorrhage ($R = -0.41$), severity and localization of subarachnoid hemorrhage ($R = -0.32$), and minimal CPP level ($R = 0.43$), on the other (Table 5.1).

Besides GCS, the significant predictive factors of outcome ($p < 0.05$) have been determined for the whole group of patients: CT categories of DAI ($R = -0.46$), degree of basal cistern compression ($R = -0.61$), severity and localization of SAH ($R = -0.40$), presence of intraventricular hemorrhage ($R = -0.43$), as well as minimal CPP level ($R = 0.34$).

Regional CBF significantly correlated with regional CBV ($R = 0.71$, $p < 0.01$); thus we analyzed only the rCBF (ml/100 g/min) parameter.

Analysis of CT perfusion data in the whole group of patients revealed the following variants of CBF: 37(92.5 %) patients had areas of rCBF reduction below 28.6 ml/100 g/min, 9 patients (22.5 %) had areas of increased rCBF over 69.0 ml/100 g/min, and 6 of these 9 patients had an increase of rCBF in one vascular region with its simultaneous reduction in the other.

It was found that rCBF parameters were higher in the middle cerebral artery (MCA) region compared to other vascular regions and subcortical formations. Thus, we have analyzed peculiarities of cerebral blood flow and its regional differences, predominant mechanisms of trauma (acceleration/deceleration, coup/contrecoup contusions, or their combinations), and predominant type of TBI (diffuse, focal, or multifocal).

Twenty-seven (67.5 %) of 40 patients sustained severe TBI in traffic accidents; therefore, the leading mechanism of brain damage was acceleration/deceleration in different combinations with coup/contrecoup impact.

All patients were divided into three groups based on the clinical signs, mechanisms of trauma, and CT data:

Group 1 included 12 (30 %) patients with DAI caused by a traffic accident.

Group 2 included 15 (37.5 %) patients with DAI in combination with cortical-subcortical contusions caused by a traffic accident, with 5 of them having epidural-subdural hematomas.

Group 3 included 13 (32.5 %) patients with brain injury resulted from a blow to the head or by the head; CT demonstrated signs of hemorrhagic or nonhemorrhagic focal contusions accompanied by epidural-subdural hematomas in 6 patients.

Table 5.1 Summarized data on clinical and instrumental studies

1	2	3	4	5	6	7	8	9	10	11	12	13	14	15	16	17
N	Age, gender	DAI category	Contusion type	Hematoma type	SAH	IVH	Midline shift	Basal cisterns	GCS	Coma duration	GOS	Min CPP	Max ICP	Ischemia, %	Hyperemia, %	Surgery type
1	18 F	3	No	–	3	1	0	3	4	6	3	55	35	37.5	0	VSH
2	23 F	3	No	–	2	0	0	3	5	11	3	60	18	50	0	
3	37 M	1	No	–	0	0	0	1	7	2	5	87	23	66	0	
4	24 M	1	No	–	2	1	0	1	5	27	3	50	40	12.5	0	
5	22 F	3	No	–	3	0	0	4	4	17	3	23	55	25	0	Rcr, L
6	17 M	1	No	–	0	0	0	3	7	3	5	65	15	0	12.5	
7	23 M	3	No	–	3	1	0	4	4	7	1	24	50	12.5	0	
8	29 M	1	No	–	0	0	0	1	7	6	4	73	16	25	0	
9	22 F	3	No	–	3	1	0	4	4	5	1	50	30	30	0	DEC R+L
10	30 M	1	No	–	0	0	0	1	7	14	4	86	15	25	12.5	
11	29 F	2	No	–	1	0	0	1	5	6	3	86	27	25	0	
12	17 F	1	No	–	0	0	0	1	7	4	4	60	20	0	25	
13	26 M	2	2	–	1	0	0	2	7	10	5	59	40	12.5	0	
14	20 M	1	2	–	2	0	0	1	7	12	4	74	26	50	0	
15	23 M	3	2	–	2	0	0	3	7	8	3	75	15	12.5	12.5	Sfr
16	34 M	3	2	SDH, R	3	0	12	3	4	8	3	67	28	25	0	DECSDHr
17	38 M	3	2	SDH, L	3	1	5	2	4	15	1	60	50	0	50	Rcr SDHr
18	37 M	1	2	SDH, L	3	0	2	1	8	11	4	95	48	75	0	
19	31 M	2	2	–	3	0	0	2	7	14	4	59	30	12.5	0	DEC L
20	51 F	3	2	–	3	1	4	3	5	10	3	55	22	25	0	DEC R, SDHr
21	16 F	2	2	SDH, R	3	1	3	2	7	7	5	50	40	25	0	
22	26 M	2	2	–	3	0	6	2	6	7	4	50	20	33	0	
23	25 M	2	2	–	3	0	5	2	8	17	3	90	28	12.5	0	
24	17 F	3	1	SDH, R	3	0	7	2	7	9	4	55	20	50	37.5	Oser SDHr
25	38 F	3	2	–	3	0	0	3	4	9	1	50	35	25	0	DEC R

(continued)

Table 5.1 (continued)

1	2	3	4	5	6	7	8	9	10	11	12	13	14	15	16	17
N	Age, gender	DAI category	Contusion type	Hematoma type	SAH	IVH	Midline shift	Basal cisterns	GCS	Coma duration	GOS	Min CPP	Max ICP	Ischemia, %	Hyperemia, %	Surgery type
26	20 M	2	2	–	3	0	5	3	5	6	4	80	32	12.5	12.5	
27	54 M	1	2	–	3	0	0	1	8	11	5	70	24	12.5	0	
28	42 F	No	3	SDH	3	0	0	3	6	9	3	30	50	12.5	37.5	DEC SDHr
29	29 M	No	2	–	3	0	2	1	8	3	5	80	27	12.5	62.5	
30	33 M	No	3	–	3	1	10	3	7	6	3	60	24	17	0	DEC L
31	48 M	No	3	–	3	0	4	2	7	13	3	30	50	25	0	DEC L, ICHr
32	29 M	No	2	SDH, L	3	0	10	4	4	8	1	70	27	66	0	DEC L, SDHr
33	25 M	No	3	–	1	0	0	1	8	7	4	70	26	17	0	
34	31 M	No	3	EDH, L	3	0	4	1	7	4	4	74	25	12.5	0	Rcr EDHr
35	28 M	No	2	–	3	0	0	1	8	3	5	87	28	12.5	0	
36	32 M	No	1	EDH, L	1	0	8	2	7	9	4	30	50	25	0	DEC EDHr
37	44 M	No	2	–	3	0	0	2	4	20	2	70	20	37.5	0	Bcr
38	48 M	No	3	–	3	0	3	2	7	9	3	79	28	25	0	
39	43 M	No	3	SDH, L	3	1	10	3	4	7	1	55	12	33	0	Rcr R, SDHr
40	49 M	No	3	–	3	0	2	2	7	3	3	65	18	25	0	
Mean value	30.7						2.5		6	9.1	3.3	62.7	29.7	25.3	6.6	
min	16						0		4	2	1	23	12	0	0	
Max	54						12		8	27	5	95	55	75	62.5	
sd	10.4						3.5		1.5	5.1	1.2	18.3	11.8	17.6	15	
m	1.6						0.5		0.2	0.8	0.2	2.9	1.9	2.8	2.4	

3 – CT categories of *LAI 1–4*, by Marshall et al. (1991)

4 – Contusion CT type: 1, low density focus; 2, hemorrhagic zones of mixed density; 3, intracerebral hematoma

5 – Hematoma type, *SDH* subdural hematoma, *EDH* epidural hematoma, *ICH* intracerebral hematoma, *R* right, *L* left

6 – Subarachnoid hemorrhage: 0, absent; 1, convex; 2, basal; 3, convex+basal

7 – Intraventricular hemorrhage: 0, absent; 1, present

8 – Midline shift, mm

9 – Basal cistern compression: 0, normal; 1, moderate narrowing; 2, asymmetric deformation; 3, severe narrowing and/or deformation; 4, nonvisualized

10 – Glasgow Coma Scale

11 – Coma duration, days

12 – Glasgow Outcome Scale

13 – Minimal cerebral perfusion pressure, mmHg

14 – Maximal intracranial pressure, mmHg

15 – Ischemia: percentage of analyzed vascular regions with rCBF $\leq$ 28.6 ml/100 g/min

16 – Hyperemia: percentage of analyzed vascular regions with rCBF > 69 ml/100 g/min

17 – Types of surgery: *VSH* ventricular shunting, *Rcr* resection craniectomy, *DEC* decompressive craniectomy, *Sfr* skull bone fragments removal, *Osc* osteoplastic craniotomy, *SDHr* subdural hematoma removal, *EDHr* epidural hematoma removal, *ICHr* intracerebral hematoma removal, *Bcr* basal cranioplasty

sd standard deviation, *m* mean error

5.2   Peculiarities of rCBF in Patients with Diffuse Axonal Injury

The peculiar feature in this group (12 cases) was the development of coma lasting 2–17 days (average 9 ± 6.7 days) since the moment of trauma in 11 of 12 patients. Only one patient had a lucid interval preceding the long-term coma. Thus, patients of this group had severe primary damage of deep hemispheric and brain stem structures leading to a long-term coma from time of trauma.

A significant correlation ($p < 0.05$) was between GCS, GOS, and the following parameters: CT categories of DAI ($R = -0.89$), presence and localization of SAH ($R = -0.98$), presence of intraventricular hemorrhage ($R = 0.67$), the degree of basal cistern compression ($R = -0.70$), maximal ICP values ($R = -0.79$), and minimal CPP values ($R = 0.70$).

An evident correlation ($p < 0.05$) was obtained between outcome by GOS and the following parameters: CT categories of DAI ($R = -0.76$), presence and localization of SAH ($R = -0.83$), presence of intraventricular hemorrhage ($R = -0.72$), the degree of basal cistern compression ($R = -0.61$), maximal ICP values ($R = -0.61$), and minimal CPP values ($R = 0.64$).

CT categories of DAI (I–III) in this group of patients correlated ($p < 0.01$) with maximal ICP values ($R = 0.58$), minimal CPP values ($R = -0.63$), GCS ($R = -0.89$), and outcome ($R = -0.76$).

It should be noted that CT in 6 of 12 patients did not reveal any signs of intracranial hemorrhages (category I of DAI); basal cisterns were normal or moderately narrowed. Five of six patients were in moderate coma (GCS of 7) at admission and one patient in deep coma (GCS of 5). These five patients showed favorable outcome (GOS of 4–5), and one patient was severely disabled (GOS of 3).

CT in the other 6 of 12 patients of this group detected different combinations of hemorrhages in the white matter, subcortical formations, and midbrain, basal, and convexital subarachnoid spaces as well as intraventricular hemorrhages. All 6 patients showed signs of severe deformation, narrowing or total compression of basal cisterns. All of them were in deep coma (GCS ≤ 5), and 4 of them had signs of decerebration. All 6 patients showed unfavorable outcome (2 patients died and 4 remained in severe disability state) (Fig. 5.1).

The analysis of rCBF showed its reduction (rCBF below 28.6 ml/100 g/min) in one or several vascular regions in 7 of 12 patients (Fig. 5.2). All of them had intracranial hypertension.

In 3 of 12 cases, hyperemia was registered in one vascular region (rCBF above 69.0 ml/100 g/min); in one of these three cases, it was combined with the oligemia area (rCBF below 28.6 ml/100 g/min). The maximal ICP level in these three patients did not exceed 20 mmHg. These three patients with normal ICP values and signs of regional hyperemia showed favorable outcome.

It was determined that rCBF average values in all vascular regions were higher (not significantly) in 6 patients with category I of DAI compared to patients with categories II–III of DAI (Fig. 5.3). In this series of patients, there were no patients with category IV of DAI.

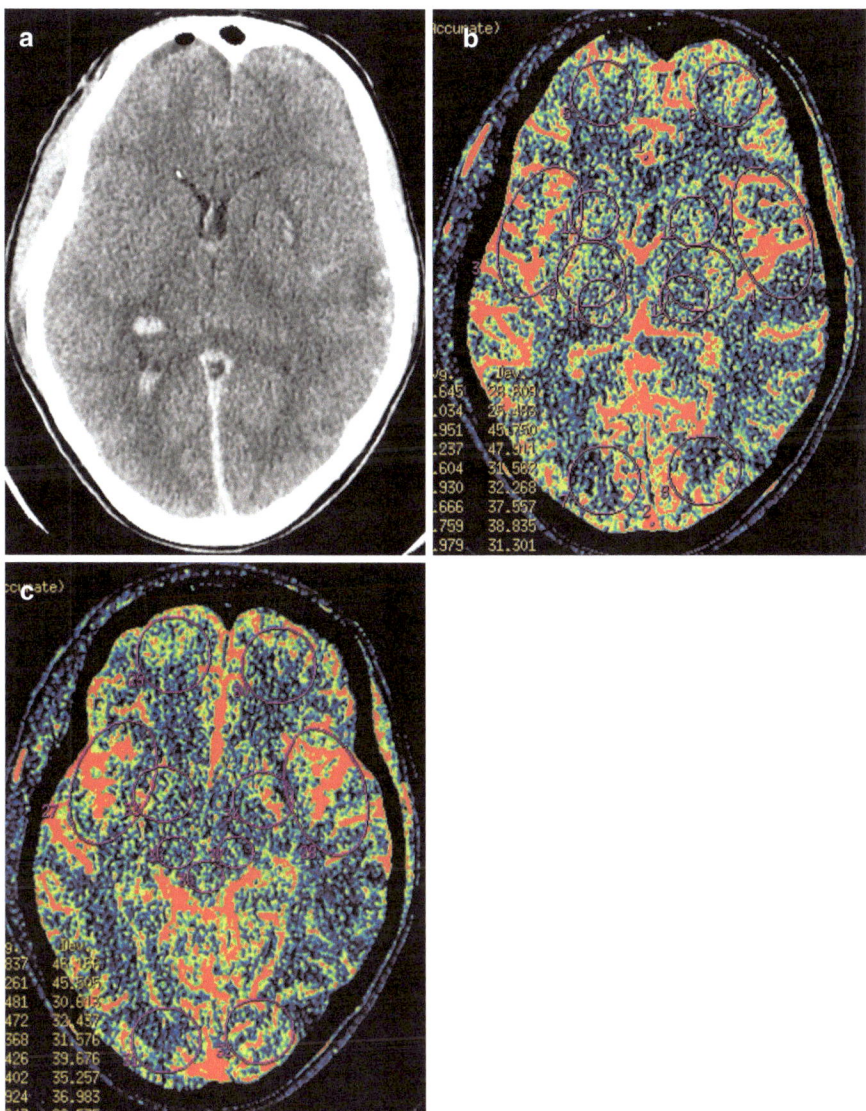

Fig. 5.1 Severe traumatic brain injury in traffic accident. GCS, 4. CT signs of DAI (**a**), multiple hemorrhagic foci in the brain parenchyma, subarachnoid and intraventricular hemorrhages, diffuse brain swelling. CT perfusion reveals blood flow parameters above 28.6 ml/100 g/min (**b, c**) in all vascular regions. Death in 5 days in the presence of unregulated intracranial hypertension

Thus, the characteristic feature of the whole group of patients with DAI was a close relationship between outcome and the following factors: presence or absence of parenchymatous, subarachnoid, and/or intraventricular hemorrhages; the degree of basal cistern compression; severity of intracranial hypertension; and presence of oligemia or ischemia combined with CPP reduction.

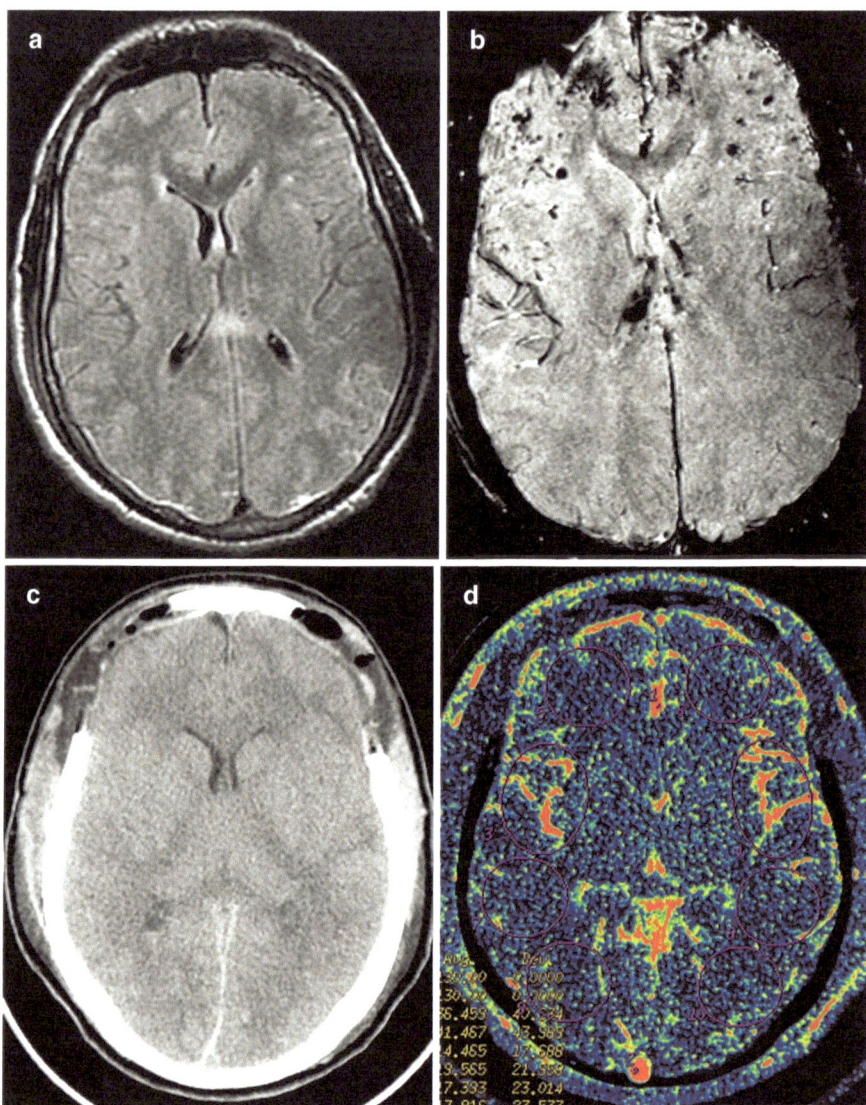

Fig. 5.2 Traffic accident. DAI. GCS, 7. Decompressive bifrontal craniectomy. Coma duration, 11 days. Outcome, moderate disability. MRI in the first day after injury (T2-FLAIR, **a**; SWAN, **b**), signs of DAI, multiple lesions of the corpus callosum, gray-white matter junction of the frontal lobes. CT (**c**); CT perfusion study (**d**) in 8 days after trauma reveals blood flow decrease in the anterior cerebral artery vascular region to 14.5 and 19.6 ml/100 g/min, in the middle and posterior cerebral artery vascular regions to 17.6 ml/100 g/min

Absolutely unfavorable prognostic factors were compression of basal cisterns, presence of hemorrhage in the midbrain, and clinical evidence of decerebration. All seven patients with these symptoms revealed different degrees of rCBF reduction in one or several vascular regions and had intracranial hypertension with subsequent unfavorable outcome (death or severe disability).

Fig. 5.3 Average rCBF values (x ± mt) in various vascular regions in different groups of patients. Significant difference of average rCBF values: *, $p < 0.01$ in vascular regions of middle cerebral arteries from ACA and PCA; **, $p < 0.05$ in subcortical formations from MCA regions; #, $p < 0.05$ in subcortical formations from ACA regions; ##, $p = 0.05$ in ACA regions in the third group of patients from the analogue values of the first group

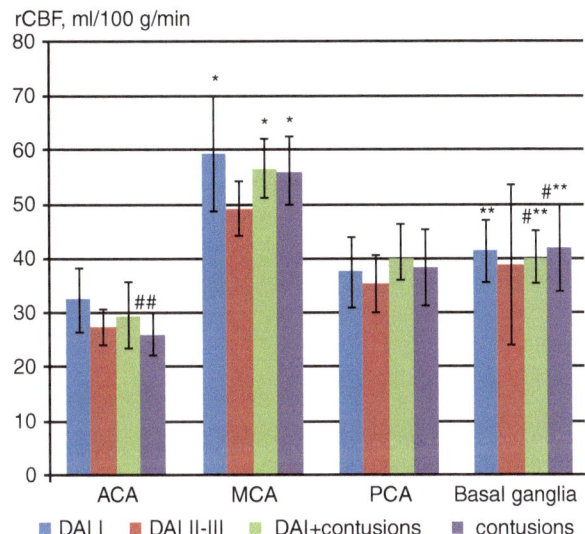

rCBF, ml/100 g/min

Legend: DAI I | DAI II-III | DAI+contusions | contusions

5.3   Peculiarities of rCBF in Patients with DAI Combined with Focal Brain Contusions

All 15 patients in this group were injured in a traffic accidents. A comatose state was developed in 11 of them immediately at the moment of trauma and lasted from 6 to 15 days. In 4 of 15 patients a lucid interval preceded coma; 5 of 15 had subdural hematomas. In 13 of 15 patients in this group, ICP was ≥ 20 mmHg.

A significant correlation ($p < 0.01$) was between GCS and the following parameters: categories of DAI ($R = -0.77$), the degree of basal cistern compression ($R = -0.62$), midline shift ($R = -0.5$), and minimal CPP values ($R = 0.6$).

An evident correlation ($p < 0.01$) was obtained between GOS and the following parameters: GCS ($R = 0.6$), CT categories of DAI ($R = -0.64$), and the degree of basal cistern compression ($R = -0.47$).

The reduction in rCBF below 28.6 ml/100 g/min in one or several vascular regions accompanied by increase of intracranial pressure (ICP > 20 mmHg) was observed in 11 of 15 patients; 4 patients had regions of elevated rCBF (rCBF > 69.0 ml/100 g/min); in 3 of them it was combined with a reduced rCBF in other vascular regions (Figs. 5.4 and 5.5).

Case Report (Fig. 5.5)

M., 28 y.o. Cause of trauma is unknown. Diagnosis: severe head injury. Subdural hematoma in the left frontotemporoparietal region. Intraventricular hemorrhage. Secondary ischemia of the brain stem and cerebral hemispheres.

On admission it is difficult to assess the patient's neurological state and level of consciousness due to sedation during transportation. Anisocoria

S > D; pupils' reaction to light is absent. Response to nociceptive stimulation – flexion of extremities and turning of the head. Cough reflex is intact.

On CT, acute subdural hematoma in the left frontotemporoparietal region. Secondary ischemia of the left hemisphere, secondary ischemic changes in vascular regions of posterior cerebral arteries on both sides. Midline shift, 8 mm. Signs of axial transtentorial dislocation.

On admission, a sudden cardiac arrest is observed. Cardiac function is restored by emergency procedures. An emergency surgery is performed: decompressive craniectomy in the left frontoparietotemporal area and removal of subdural hematoma.

In the postoperative period, GCS, 3; anisocoria S > D; pupils are of medium size; their reaction to light is absent; corneal reflex is preserved on the right, absent on the left; oculocephalic and cough reflexes are absent. On EEG recordings electrical brain activity is absent. Despite increasing doses of catecholamines, hemodynamics is unstable.

On CT in 2 days after trauma, wide areas of secondary ischemia in the brain hemispheres, subcortical formations, and brain stem. Midbrain structures are not shifted. Mesencephalic cistern is not visualized. Hemorrhagic focal contusion is in the left temporo-occipital area. Intraventricular hemorrhage is marked. CT shows descending transtentorial herniation.

Cerebral blood flow passively follows arterial pressure changes, and rCBF values in the vascular regions are as follows: for MCA regions under 80–98 ml/100 g/min, for ACA regions under 73.6–82.6 ml/100 g/min, and for the focal contusion in the left temporo-occipital region under 16.9 ml/100 g/min.

Outcome: death on the 4th day after trauma.

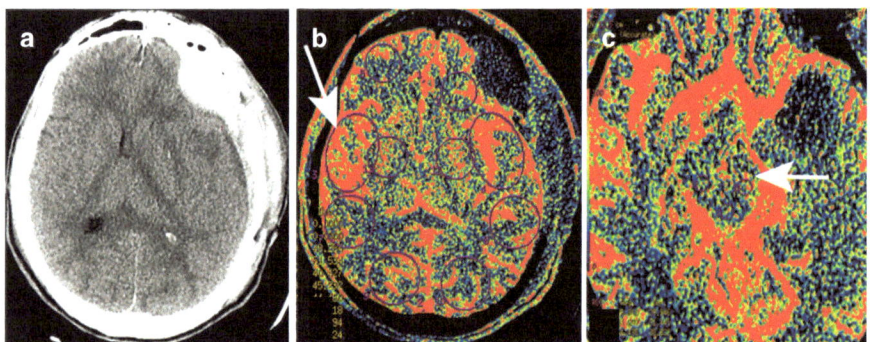

Fig. 5.4 M., 20 y.o. Severe TBI in traffic accident. GCS, 5. CT after partial removal of epidural hematoma in the left frontotemporal region (**a**). Perfusion CT study (**b, c**) reveals areas of hyperemia in the right middle cerebral artery vascular region, left cerebral peduncle (*white arrows*). Regional CBF values in the right temporal lobe, under 84.3 ml/100 g/min (normal range, 28.6–69.0 ml/100 g/min); in the left cerebral peduncle, under 51.4 ml/100 g/min (normal range, our data, 18.0–38.0 ml/100 g/min)

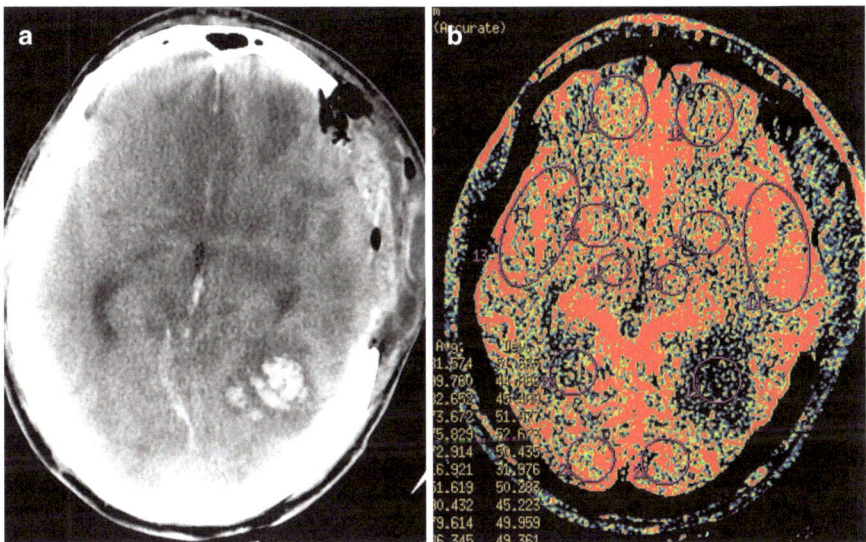

Fig. 5.5 M., 28 y.o. Focal and diffuse brain injury. GCS, 3. Decompressive craniectomy. CT (**a**); CT perfusion study (**b**) in 3 days after trauma, focal ischemia in combination with diffuse hyperemia and failure of the mechanisms of autoregulation

At the same time, mean rCBF values in the analyzed vascular territories did not significantly differ from the analogous in the previous group (with DAI only).

Two patients in deep coma (GCS of 4) showed areas of hyperemia in vascular regions at the removed subdural hematoma site. One of these patients recovered to moderate disability, the other died in 15 days following trauma due to development of extracranial and systemic complications. Two other patients revealed hyperemia in the MCA region with a simultaneous reduction of rCBF in other vascular regions.

The following prognostic factors were associated with unfavorable outcome, besides TBI severity: hemorrhagic nature of DAI, the degree of basal cistern compression, and signs of brain compression requiring surgical intervention.

5.4   Peculiarities of rCBF in Patients with Focal Brain Contusions

All 13 patients in this group had TBI caused by a blow to the head or by the head; 5 of them developed coma immediately after trauma (length of coma 7–20 days); 8 patients (length of coma 3–8 days) developed coma after a lucid interval.

CT scans revealed cortical-subcortical hemorrhagic contusions, predominantly in the frontal and temporal lobes (Fig. 5.6) and rarely in the parietal and occipital lobes. Four of them had intracranial hematomas requiring surgical intervention. According to ICP monitoring data, 11 of 13 patients showed the signs of intracranial hypertension (ICP > 20 mmHg).

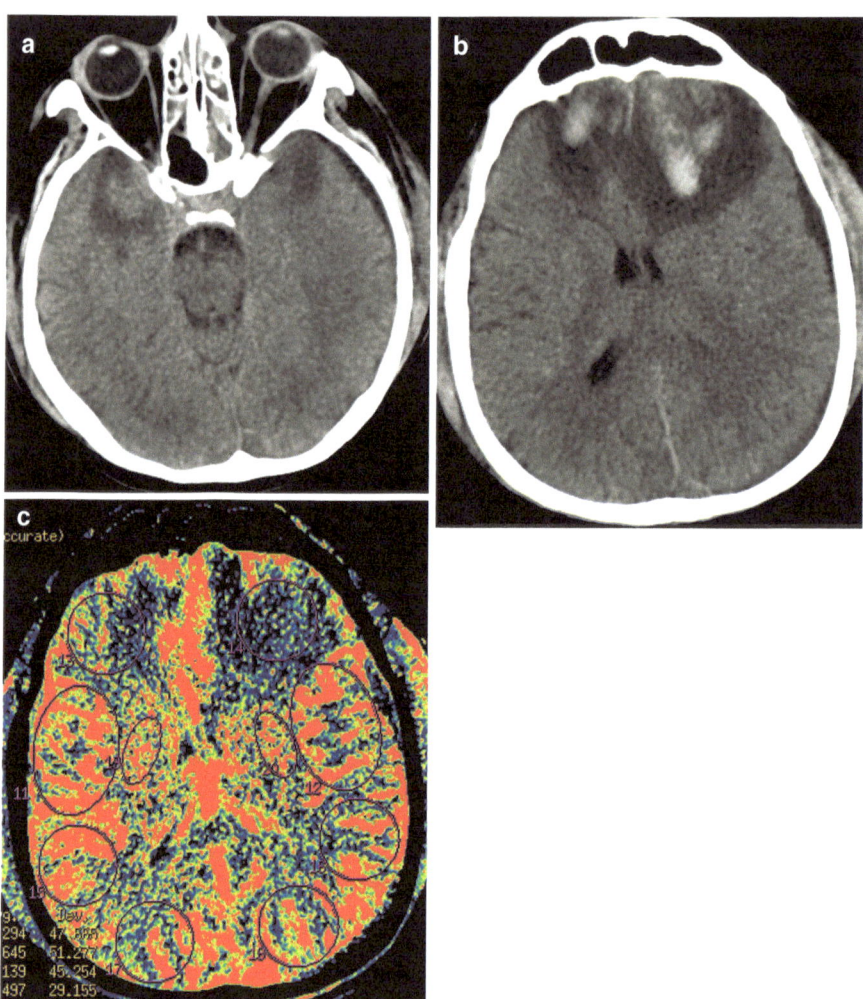

Fig. 5.6 Severe TBI caused by assault. Coma (GCS, 8) after a lucid interval. CT, signs of focal contusions in the frontal and temporal lobes (**a**, **b**). rCBF map (**c**) shows blood flow reduction in contusion areas

A significant correlation ($p<0.01$) was found between GCS and the following criteria: coma duration ($R=-0.55$), the degree of basal cistern compression ($R=-0.72$), midline shift ($R=-0.4$), percentage of vascular regions with a reduced rCBF <28.6 ml/100 g/min ($R=-0.77$), and presence of intracranial hematomas requiring surgery ($R=-0.47$).

The prognostic factors of unfavorable outcome ($p<0.05$) for this group of patients were GCS ($R=0.91$), coma duration ($R=-0.46$), midline shift ($R=-0.52$), compression of basal cisterns ($R=-0.82$), and percentage of vascular regions with rCBF reduction below 28.6 ml/100 g/min.

Mean rCBF values in ACA regions in this group of patients with focal lesions were significantly lower compared to analogous regions in patients with DAI only. It was due to predominating focal lesions in the frontal lobes in these patients (Fig. 5.3).

5.5   Peculiarities of rCBF in the Contusion Areas

Perfusion studies showed that cerebral blood flow values in contusions were 16.3 ± 6 ml/100 g/min, while in the analogous intact structures of the opposite hemisphere, they were significantly higher (36.0 ± 10 ml/100 g/min, $p < 0.01$).

On the whole, 27 of 28 patients (96 %) with severe TBI and brain contusions had rCBF values below 28.6 ml/100 g/min in one and more vascular regions; only 6 (21 %) patients had rCBF over 69.0 ml/100 g/min, thus indicating regional hyperemia, and in five of them it was combined with oligemia or ischemia in the other vascular regions.

5.6   Study of rCBF in Subcortical Formations (Basal Ganglia and Thalami)

According to our research, mean rCBF values in subcortical formations did not significantly differ from the analogous values in the region of middle cerebral arteries (MCA) and were distinct from the values obtained in the territories of anterior (ACA) and especially in posterior cerebral arteries (PCA). These differences can be explained by various proportions of the white and gray matter in the analyzed region of interest (ROI), as well as by large vessel involvement. There were no significant differences between mean rCBF values in subcortical formations in groups of patients with predominant diffuse or focal brain contusions.

Figure 5.1 (patient 9, Table 5.1) shows the CT perfusion study in territories of anterior, middle, and posterior cerebral arteries and selectively in the basal ganglia, thalami, and midbrain in a patient in deep coma (GCS, 4). She had hemorrhagic type of DAI; intracerebral, subarachnoid, and intraventricular hemorrhages; severe diffuse brain volume enlargement; and narrowing of the ventricular system and basal cisterns. rCBF values in the basic vascular regions and subcortical formations were ranged from 28.6 to 69.0 ml/100 g/min. It should be mentioned that CT perfusion in this patient was performed in the first 24 h after TBI and with the diffuse brain edema being present. Further increasing of edema and intracranial hypertension resulted in death on the fifth day after trauma.

5.7   Discussion

Our studies showed that the three examined groups of patients with a relatively similar severity of TBI (GCS of ≤ 8 at admission) had different variants of brain damage (DAI $\pm$ focal contusions $\pm$ intracranial hematomas), as well as different CPP and rCBF response (Potapov et al. 2011). The dominating mechanism of TBI in 27 of 40 patients (67.5 %) was acceleration-deceleration (traffic accidents) which usually resulted in DAI of different severity with or without focal contusions.

The most significant characteristics of trauma severity for the whole group of patients, besides GCS, were development of long-term coma since the moment of trauma, CT features of the basal cistern compression, presence of intraventricular hemorrhage and subarachnoid hemorrhage, as well as low minimal values of cerebral perfusion pressure.

The data obtained have confirmed the clinical and predictive value of brain displacement in neurosurgical pathology earlier described in details by Blinkov and Smirnov (1967) in their clinical and morphological studies and later on in studies devoted to comparison of clinical and CT data in TBI (Potapov 1989, 2003; Zakharova 2000; Wintermark et al. 2001; Kornienko et al. 2003; Kornienko and Pronin 2009; Maas et al. 2005; Saatman et al. 2008). Intracranial hemorrhages, development of focal, hemispheric, or diffuse edema and ischemia, and brain swelling caused by hyperemia lead to disturbance of the relationship between intracranial volume and pressure followed by lateral and axial shift of the brain. It was determined that the degree of basal cistern compression as an indicator of CSF space depletion was a significant predictive criterion correlating with CPP.

The results of cerebral blood flow study in hemispheric structures showed that rCBF values were below 28.6 ml/100 g/min in 37 of 40 examined patients. In 9 patients only they were over 69 ml/100 g/min. This range of rCBF values for a preliminary analysis served as an indicator of oligemia or hyperemia. It was earlier obtained by Wintermark et al. (2004a, b) using CT perfusion in 32 control subjects and reflected average rCBF±2 standard deviations. Application of this range as "normal" in our study might be explained by only a few publications studying rCBF in healthy volunteers (Pronin et al. 2007). At the same time, the experience gained by using CT perfusion has shown dependence of the values of three blood flow parameters (rCBF, rCBV, and MTT) upon the following aspects:

• Choice of a region of interest (ROI) with predominant gray and white matter as well as large vessel involvement
• Presence of signs of brain structure damage, hemorrhage, edema, etc., in the regions of interest

Our results showed that average rCBF values in the regions of MCA were significantly higher compared to other vascular regions (ACA and PCA) and subcortical structures in all analyzed groups of patients.

This may serve as a reason to standardize ROIs in different vascular regions when evaluating cerebral blood flow levels. In our opinion, such an approach is justified because it allows a better understanding of severe diffuse axonal and focal brain injury pathogenesis.

It was determined that 3 of 6 patients with nonhemorrhagic DAI revealed high CBF values in one or two MCA regions with the maximal ICP values not exceeding 20 mmHg. Similarly, increased ICP values (>25 mmHg) were observed in 5 of 6 patients with hemorrhagic DAI, and one patient had normal ICP. All 6 patients with hemorrhagic DAI and cerebral blood flow disturbances developed unfavorable outcome: severe disability (4) or death (2).

The most significant predictive factors for the group of patients with DAI ($n = 12$) were GCS, maximal values of ICP, minimal values of CPP, severity of SAH, presence of intraventricular hemorrhage, and degree of basal cistern compression.

Combination of CT signs of DAI and focal contusions was observed in 15 of 27 patients injured in a traffic accident; 5 of them had subdural hematomas. A significant correlation was found in this group between trauma severity (GCS) and CT categories of DAI, signs of brain compression, and midline shift. In 11 of 15 patients a reduction in rCBF values in one or several vascular regions was detected, and only 4 patients had signs of regional hyperemia.

There were found correlations between severity and outcome of trauma, on the one hand, and length of coma, midline shift, and brain stem structure compression, on the other, in patients with predominant brain contusions. All patients in this group had oligemic or ischemic areas in one or more vascular regions, and in two of them CT perfusion showed signs of hyperemia in other vascular regions.

rCBF values in hemorrhagic supratentorial contusions of mixed density (16.3 ± 6 ml/100 g/min) were close to those in hemorrhagic contusion foci (9.2 ± 6.6 ml/100 g/min) obtained by Soustiel et al. (2008) using CT perfusion and to those in the ischemic zones (14.0 ± 9 ml/100 g/min) obtained by Wintermark et al. (2001) by both CT perfusion and xenon-enhanced CT methods in the same patients.

Regional hypoperfusion (oligemia) or ischemia in severe TBI can be caused by the following factors: angiospasm resulting from SAH, brain edema, intracranial hypertension, autoregulation disturbances associated with episodes of CPP decrease, and direct impact on the vessels. In our series of patients, each of these factors and their combinations could be the reason for rCBF decrease and brain ischemia.

In our study, rCBF values have been obtained for the first time both in the main vascular regions and selectively in the basal ganglia and thalami using CT perfusion in patients with severe diffuse and focal brain injuries.

The regional or diffuse brain hyperemia in patients with severe TBI was probably caused by failure of the mechanisms of autoregulation, venous outflow disturbance, tissue acidosis, hypermetabolism, convulsions, hypercapnia, or hypoxia (Lassen 1966; Lassen and Christenson 1976; Maksakova 1978; Bruce et al. 1981; Mendelow and Teasdale 1983; Glazman et al. 1988; Potapov 1989; Reilly and Bullock 2005; Wintermark et al. 2006).

All our patients were in coma during the CT perfusion study. They all had artificial ventilation with normal arterial blood of pO_2 and pCO_2. For this reason, we did not regard hypercapnia and hypoxemia as a cause of regional hyperemia which was observed in 9 of 40 patients. The necessity of using a subnarcotic dosage of propofol or benzodiazepine for synchronizing artificial ventilation is unlikely to result in cerebral hypermetabolism and be the cause of regional blood flow increase. There are reasons to suggest that regional hyperemia in these patients should be caused by rCBF regulation disorders or cerebral venous outflow impairment (Potapov et al. 2011). Our hypothesis was proved by the fact that three of our patients with signs of regional hyperemia showed minimal CPP values above 75 mmHg, while in the other two patients, regional hyperemia was observed after removal of subdural hematoma and decompressive craniectomy. In such cases we may deal with disordered cerebral blood flow autoregulation with increased CPP values and postischemic hyperemia or reperfusion after brain decompression (Zakharova 2013).

In our series of patients with severe TBI, we revealed a great variety of primary focal and diffuse brain damages and parenchymatous, subarachnoid, and epidural-subdural hemorrhages underlying a wide spectrum of secondary pathophysiological mechanisms (development of edema, disturbances of intracranial volume and pressure relationship, cerebral perfusion pressure, etc.). Under these conditions, the most important data for an adequate assessment of TBI severity, its pathophysiology, as well as prognosis of the time course and outcome were mechanisms of trauma, dynamics of patients' clinical condition, as well as results of complex diagnosis of focal, multifocal, and/or diffuse brain lesions and hemorrhages and midbrain and brain stem shifts and compressions. Intracranial hypertension with reduced CBF and CPP is considered the predominant pathophysiological phenomenon of severe TBI.

Secondary mechanisms of brain damage have proved to be the cause of coma development after a lucid interval in one third of our patients and unfavorable outcome – in half of them. rCBF increase in one vascular region with its decrease in the other, observed in some of our patients, did not permit us to recommend any universal algorithm for a vasoactive treatment of severe TBI.

There is a strong need for further studying of pathogenesis of different variants of cerebral blood flow changes, their relationship with ICP and CPP dynamics. Special emphasis should be placed on localization and severity of pathological changes verified by modern methods of neuroimaging.

References

Blinkov S, Smirnov N (1967) Brain displacement and deformations. Medicine, Leningrad

Bruce D, Alavi A, Bilamut M et al (1981) Diffuse cerebral swelling following head injuries in children: the syndrome of malignant brain edema. J Neurosurg 54(1):170–178

Glazman L, Potapov A, Tomas J (1988) Hemispheric cerebral blood flow in different types of traumatic brain injury. Zh Vopr Neurokhir Im N N Burdenko 4:35–39

Kornienko V, Pronin I (eds) (2009) Diagnostic Neuroradiology. Springer-Verlag: Berlin Heidelberg

Kornienko V, Potapov A, Pronin I, Zakharova N (2003) Diagnostic possibilities of computed and magnetic resonance imaging in traumatic brain injury. In: Potapov A, Likhterman L, Zelman V et al (eds) Evidence-based neurotraumatology. Andreeva TM: Moscow, pp 408–461

Lassen N (1966) The luxury perfusion syndrome and its possible relationship to acute metabolic acidosis localized within the brain. Lancet 2:1113–1116

Lassen N, Christenson M (1976) Physiology of cerebral blood flow. Br J Anaesth 48:719–734

Maas A, Hukkelhoven C, Marshall L et al (2005) Prediction of outcome in traumatic brain injury with computed tomographic characteristics a comparison between the computed tomographic classification and combinations of computed tomographic predictors. Neurosurgery 57: 1173–1182

Maksakova O (1978) Adequate cerebral blood flow disturbances in coma states in neurosurgical clinical practice. Dissertation, Burdenko Neurosurgery Institute, Moscow

Marshall L, Marshall S, Klauber M, Clark M (1991) A new classification of head injury based on computerized tomography. J Neurosurg 75:14–20

Mendelow A, Teasdale G (1983) Pathophysiology of head injuries. Br J Surg 70(11):641–650

Potapov A (1989) Pathogenesis and differentiated treatment of focal and diffuse brain injuries. Dissertation, Kiev Neurosurgical Institute

Potapov A, Likhterman L, Zelman V, Kornienko V, Kravchuk A (eds) (2003) Evidence-based neurotraumatology. Andreeva TM: Moscow

Potapov A, Zakharova N, Pronin I et al (2011) Prognostic value of ICP, CPP and regional blood flow monitoring in diffuse and focal traumatic cerebral lesions. Zh Vopr Neirokhir Im N N Burdenko 75(3):3–16

Pronin I, Fadeeva L, Zakharova N, Dolgushin M, Kornienko V (2007) Perfusion CT: evaluation of cerebral blood flow in normal subject. Med Visualiz 3:8–12

Reilly P, Bullock R (2005) Head injury – pathophysiology and management, 2nd edn. Hodder Arnold, London

Saatman K, Duhaime A, Bullock R et al (2008) Classification of traumatic brain injury for targeted therapies. J Neurotrauma 25:719–728

Soustiel J, Mahamid E, Goldsher D, Zaaroor M (2008) Perfusion –CT for early assessment of traumatic cerebral contusion. Neuroradiology 50:189–196

Teasdale G, Jennett B (1974) Assessment of coma and impaired consciousness. A practical scale. Lancet 2:81–85

Wintermark M, Thiran J, Maeder P et al (2001) Simultaneous measurements of regional cerebral blood flow by perfusion-CT and stable xenon-CT: a validation study. AJNR Am J Neuroradiol 22:905–914

Wintermark M, Chiolero R, van Melle G et al (2004a) Relationship between brain perfusion computed tomography variables and cerebral perfusion pressure in severe head trauma patients. Clin Care Med 32(7):1579–1587

Wintermark M, van Melle G, Schnyder P et al (2004b) Admission perfusion CT: prognostic value in patients with severe head trauma. Radiology 232:211–220

Wintermark M, Chiolero R, van Melle G et al (2006) Cerebral vascular autoregulation assessed by perfusion-CT in severe head trauma patients. J Neuroradiol 33:27–37

Zakharova N (2000) Clinical and prognostic value of brain displacement and deformation in the acute period of traumatic brain injury. Dissertation, Voronezh State Medical Academy

Zakharova N (2013) Neuroimaging of structural and hemodynamic disturbances in severe traumatic brain injury (clinical CT – MRI studies). Dissertation, Burdenko Neurosurgery Institute, Moscow

Dynamics of Hemispheric and Brain Stem Regional Cerebral Blood Flow

6

Contents

6.1   Clinical Material   125
6.2   Dynamics of rCBF in Hemispheric Brain Structures   126
6.3   Analysis of rCBF in the Brain Stem   138
6.4   Dynamic Studies of rCBF in the Brain Stem..   141
6.5   Discussion...   146
References...   153

6.1   Clinical Material

24 patients with TBI caused by a traffic accident (13), blow to the head (7), falls from height (3), and blind penetrating wound (1) were included into the analysis. Patients' age ranged 6–49 (average 32.5 ± 13), 16 of them were male and 8 female; 21 patients had an admission Glasgow Coma Scale (GCS) score of 4–8 (6.4 ± 1.5) and 3 patients had GCS of 9–11. Dynamic evaluation revealed that 21 patients had length of coma ranging 3–20 days (average 9.8 ± 4 days); 10 patients had a lucid interval after trauma.

On admission CT data analysis revealed cortical-subcortical contusions in 22 cases, signs of diffuse brain injury in 11 cases. All patients showed CT signs of subarachnoid hemorrhage and different degrees of compression or deformation of mesencephalic cisterns, and 10 patients had a lateral midbrain shift. Outcome analysis by GOS showed that only 10 (42 %) patients had favorable outcome (moderate disability or good recovery), 14 (58 %) unfavorable outcome: severe disability (11), vegetative state (1), and death (2).

The first rCBF study was performed within the first 1–3 days following TBI in 12 patients, within 4–8 days in 8 patients, and within 12–14 days in 4 patients. The second rCBF evaluation was performed within 5–14 days after trauma in 14 patients, within 15–34 days in 9 patients, and on the 60th day in one patient. Regional CBF was evaluated four times in one patient – the third and fourth studies were

---

This chapter has been contributed in collaboration with Eugenia Alexandrova and Gleb Danilov.

N. Zakharova et al., *Neuroimaging of Traumatic Brain Injury*,
DOI 10.1007/978-3-319-04355-5_6, © Springer International Publishing Switzerland 2014

performed in 4 and 6 months following TBI due to development of hydrocephalus. In another patient CT perfusion was carried out three times; the last one in 7 months after trauma and shunting procedure following cranioplasty.

Twenty patients with severe TBI in coma and 4 patients with mild TBI underwent a single CT perfusion study with blood flow evaluations in the brain stem, and 18 patients underwent CT perfusion study in dynamics with ROIs positioning at the region of the midbrain tegmentum and in both cerebral peduncles symmetrically.

Four healthy volunteers without history of a neurological disease or significant head trauma were studied using the same CT perfusion parameters; age range was 21–36 (mean = 30) (Pronin et al. 2007).

6.2   Dynamics of rCBF in Hemispheric Brain Structures

Perfusion CT studies demonstrated average rCBF values exceeding 28.6–69.0 ml/100 g/min in single or multiple vascular regions in 23 patients, with seven of them showing rCBF reduction in one or more vascular regions and its increase in the other regions. A significant correlation was identified between regional cerebral blood flow (rCBF) and cerebral blood volume (rCBV) values ($R = 0.8$, $p < 0.05$). For these reasons further analysis was based on rCBF values only.

The lowest rCBF values were obtained in the vascular regions of ACA in the first studies and the following days and weeks after trauma. This tendency toward rCBF reduction in the ACA regions was caused by predominant frontal lobe contusions. Typical rCBF maps are presented in Fig. 6.1. A comparison analysis showed a significant difference ($p < 0.05$) between average rCBF values in hemorrhagic contusions and in the contralateral hemispheric intact zones.

CT scanning in two patients in deep coma at admission (GCS of 4) showed signs of diffuse and focal brain injury followed by hydrocephalus (Figs. 6.2 and 6.3).

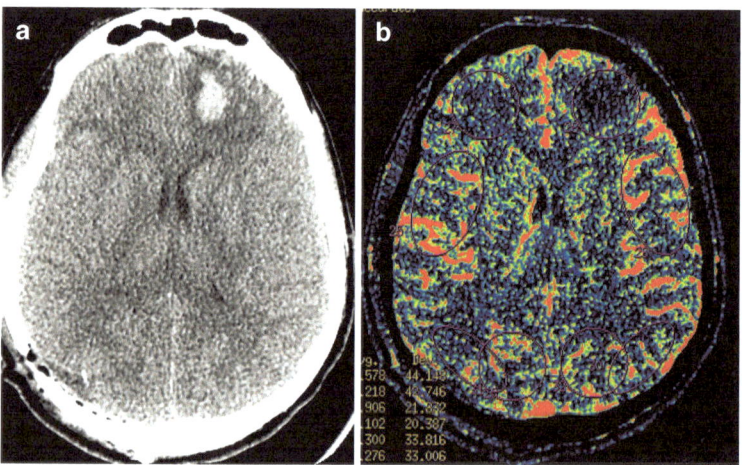

Fig. 6.1 Traumatic brain injury as a result of fall from height. GCS, 7. Outcome, severe disability. Focal contusions of the frontal and temporal lobes. Cerebral perfusion study in 2 (**a, b**) and 10 (**c, d**) days after injury and after removal of epidural hematoma in the right parieto-occipital region; rCBF values in the focal contusion area of the left frontal lobe – 8.5 ml/100 g/min

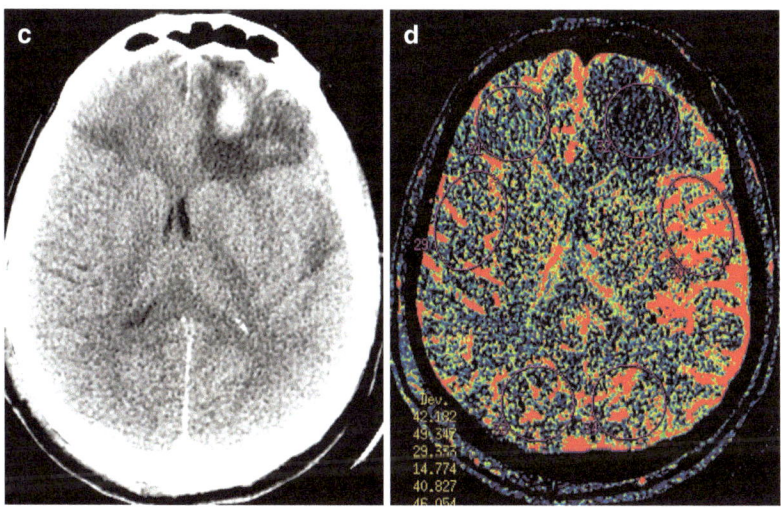

Fig. 6.1 (continued)

Case Report (Fig. 6.2)

M., 44y.o. Trauma is caused by assault. Diagnosis: diffuse axonal injury combined with hemorrhagic focal contusions in the frontal lobes, epidural hematoma in the left temporal region, linear fractures of the right frontotemporal area, frontal squama spreading into frontal sinus walls, maxillary fracture by type Le Fort II, fractures of lateral and medial walls of both orbits, zygomatic arch on the right, bilateral eye contusion.

On admission: GCS, 4; all brain stem reflexes were decreased, decerebrate rigidity.

Regional CBF values on the 5th day after trauma were 28.5 and 27.0 ml/100 g/min in the left and right ACA regions, correspondingly.

In 2 weeks after TBI, brain stem reflex is activated (blinks, "hippus pupillare," intact cough reflex, slight horizontal left eye movements).

In 25 days after TBI, osteoplastic craniotomy with plasty of the anterior skull base CSF fistula and removal of chronic subdural hematoma were performed.

In a month after TBI, patient's state is assessed as vegetative: spontaneous eye opening, oromandibular activity, decreased diffuse muscle tone are preserved. Mostly upper brain stem signs are marked.

In 40 days after TBI, clinical signs of infectious purulent meningitis confirmed by clinical and laboratory data. In 2 months after TBI, meningitis completely regressed; neurological status remains unchanged.

Dynamic CT scans in 2.5 months after TBI revealed increasing hydrocephalus, atrophic changes in frontal lobes. The patient underwent ventriculoperitoneal shunting.

Perfusion CT in a month after TBI revealed rCBF decrease to 14.4 and 10.6 ml/100 g/min, and in 6 months to 7.8 and 10.6 ml/100 g/min in the ACA territories.

In 19 months after TBI in neurological status, akinetic mutism with some emotional reactions, long-term gaze fixation, sitting in bed (for an hour), looking onto the street. Spastic tetraparesis is retained.

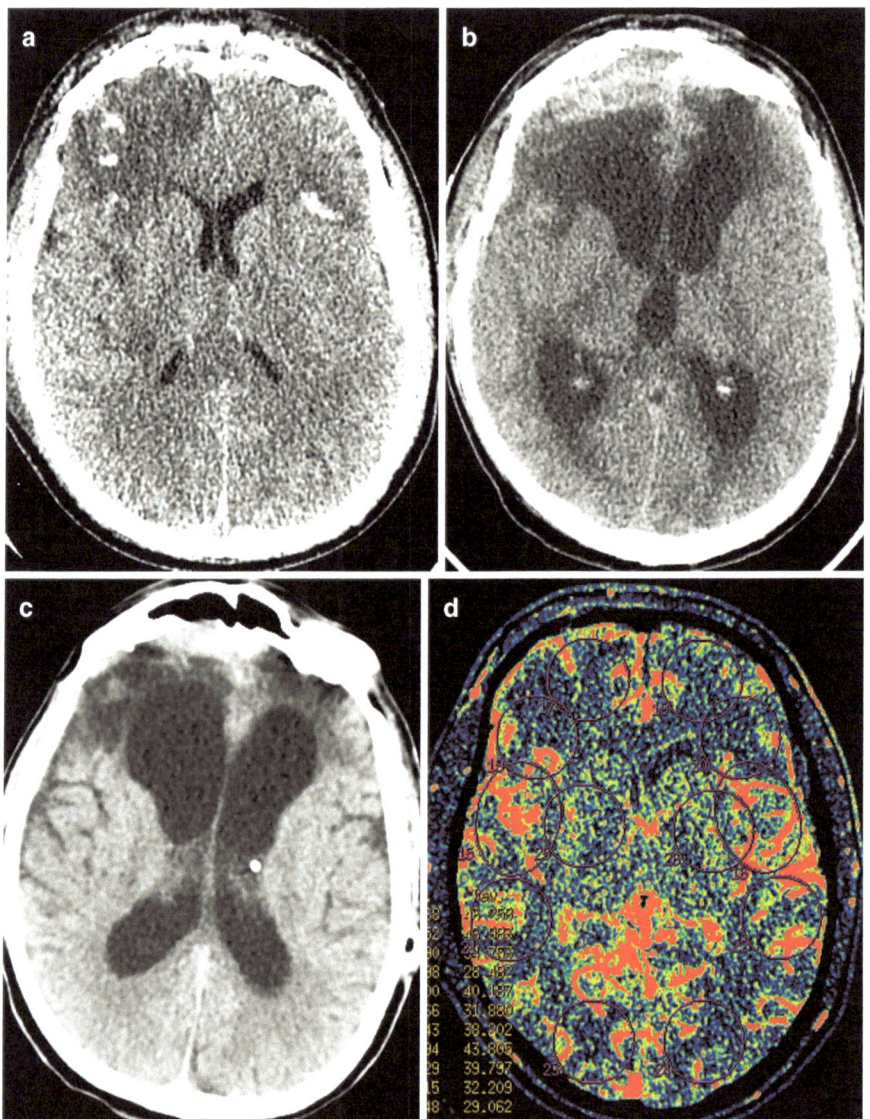

Fig. 6.2 Diffuse axonal injury with focal contusions in the frontal lobe, skull base fractures with a CSF leakage complicated by meningoencephalitis and hydrocephalus. CT and CT perfusion: (**a, d**) 5 days after injury; GCS, 4; (**b, e**) 1 month after trauma, vegetative state; (**c, f**) 6 months after injury, vegetative state (*see explanation in the text*)

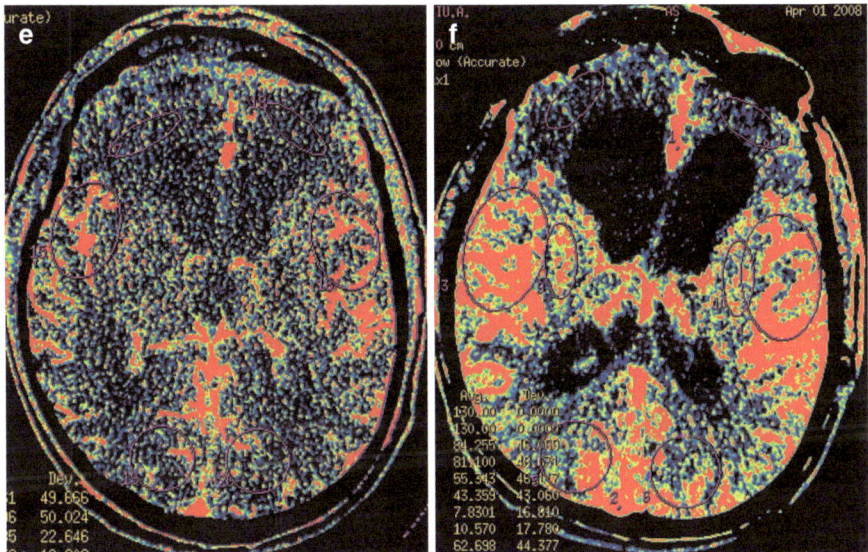

Fig. 6.2   (continued)

The other patient had diffuse and focal brain injury caused by a car accident and was in a deep coma at admission (GCS of 4). On the 2nd day following trauma, rCBF values in the right ACA region were reduced to 17.8 ml/100 g/min (and 28.2 ml/100 g/min – in the left ACA region). On the 4th day patient's state deteriorated: there were clinical and CT data of brain dislocation. For these reasons, a right-sided decompressive craniectomy was performed which allowed stabilizing patient's state and minimizing signs of brain shift and herniation. However, the patient remained in a comatose state. Repeated CT perfusion on the 11th day following trauma showed further reduction of rCBF values in both ACA artery regions (7.7 and 15.9 ml/100 g/min, accordingly) (Fig. 6.3). Later on, the comatose state was followed by the vegetative state with development of hydrocephalus which required programmable shunt implantation. The patient's state slightly improved. He showed signs of partial consciousness recovery with further transformation into minimally conscious state. Control CT studies in 4 and 7 months after trauma demonstrated signs of moderate brain atrophy (mostly in the right hemisphere) with retained rCBF reduction in the right and left ACA regions – 13.4 and 24.4 ml/100 g/min, correspondingly.

Figure 6.4 shows MRI and perfusion CT data in a patient aged 16, with epidural hematoma and contusion foci in the right temporoparietal region before and after hematoma removal. As is clear from this picture, dynamic examinations visualized the decreased edema and oligemic areas after surgery.

When focal contusions were accompanied by persistent or increasing ischemia, dynamic CT perfusion studies revealed development of cystic-atrophic changes (Fig. 6.5).

Regional CBF increase over 69.0 ml/100 g/min in the MCA vascular region was revealed in 6 patients by initial examination (3–4 days after trauma). Repeated CT perfusion studies (8–13 days after injury) in 3 of them showed preserved rCBF elevation in these vascular regions.

Figure 6.6 shows rCBF dynamics in a patient aged 49 on the 4th and 13th day after injury and subdural hematoma removal in the left frontotemporoparietal

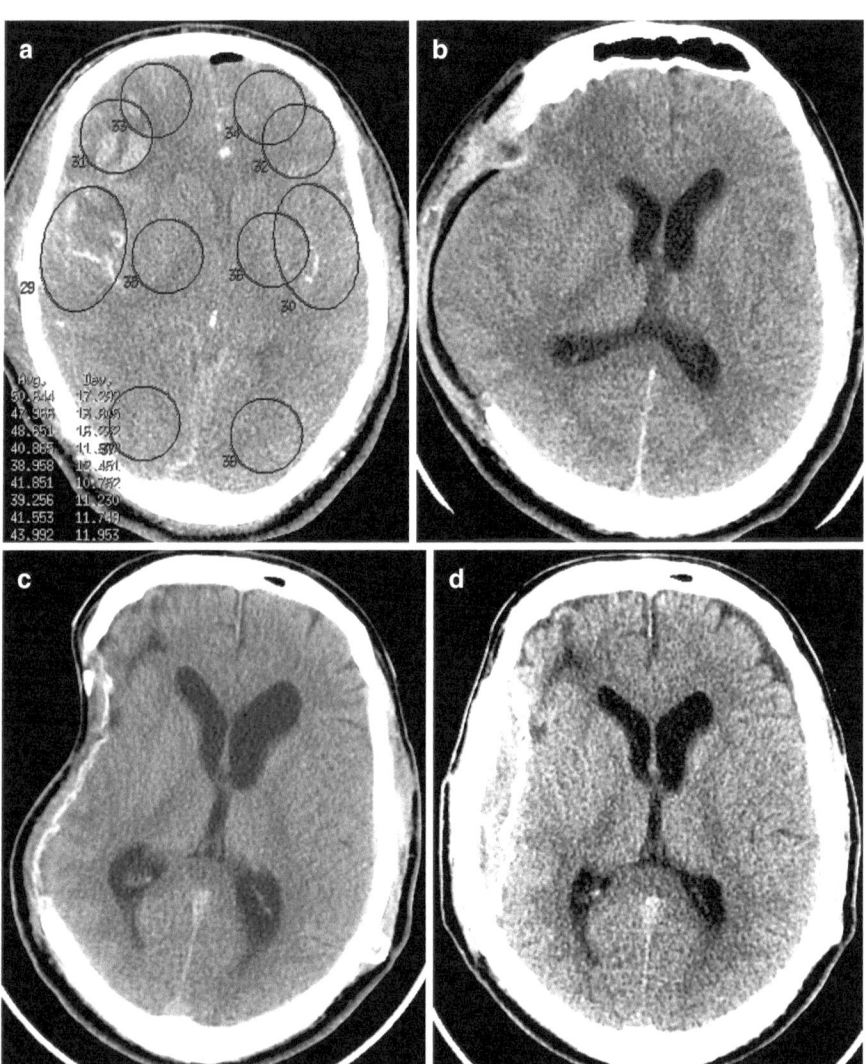

Fig. 6.3 TBI in traffic accident, DAI. GCS, 4. CT and CT perfusion: (**a, e**) (2 days after trauma), coma, decompressive craniectomy; (**b, f**) 11 days after trauma, coma, vegetative state; (**c, g**) 4 months after trauma, minimally conscious state, shunting; (**d, h**) 7 months, severe disability, cranioplasty (*see explanation in the text*)

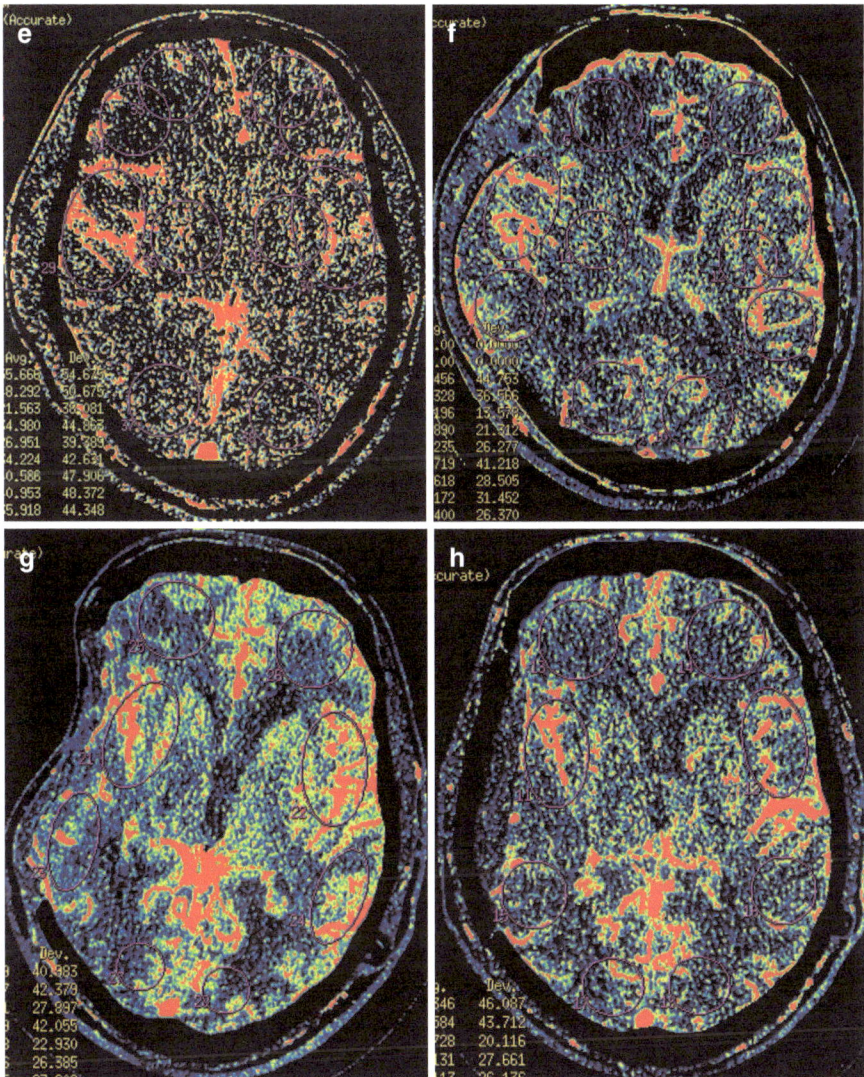

Fig.6.3 (continued)

region. It visualized rCBF value reduction (below 7.4 ml/100 g/min) in frontal, temporal, and parietal focal contusions in the left hemisphere and rCBF values increase (82.4 ml/100 g/min) in the right MCA region. A repeated CT perfusion study on the 13th day following trauma demonstrated decreased area of hemorrhage and slight regress of perifocal edema and oligemia in the contusion foci. Hyperemia was also decreased in the right MCA region. However, in 6 months following trauma, the patient remained severely disabled with aphasia and right-sided hemiparesis.

We revealed a persistent rCBF increase in the right MCA and ACA regions after removal of subdural hematoma in the right frontotemporal region in a patient aged 17 who sustained brain injury in a car accident. She had a lucid interval with further development of a moderate coma (GCS score 7; coma duration, 9 days) followed by

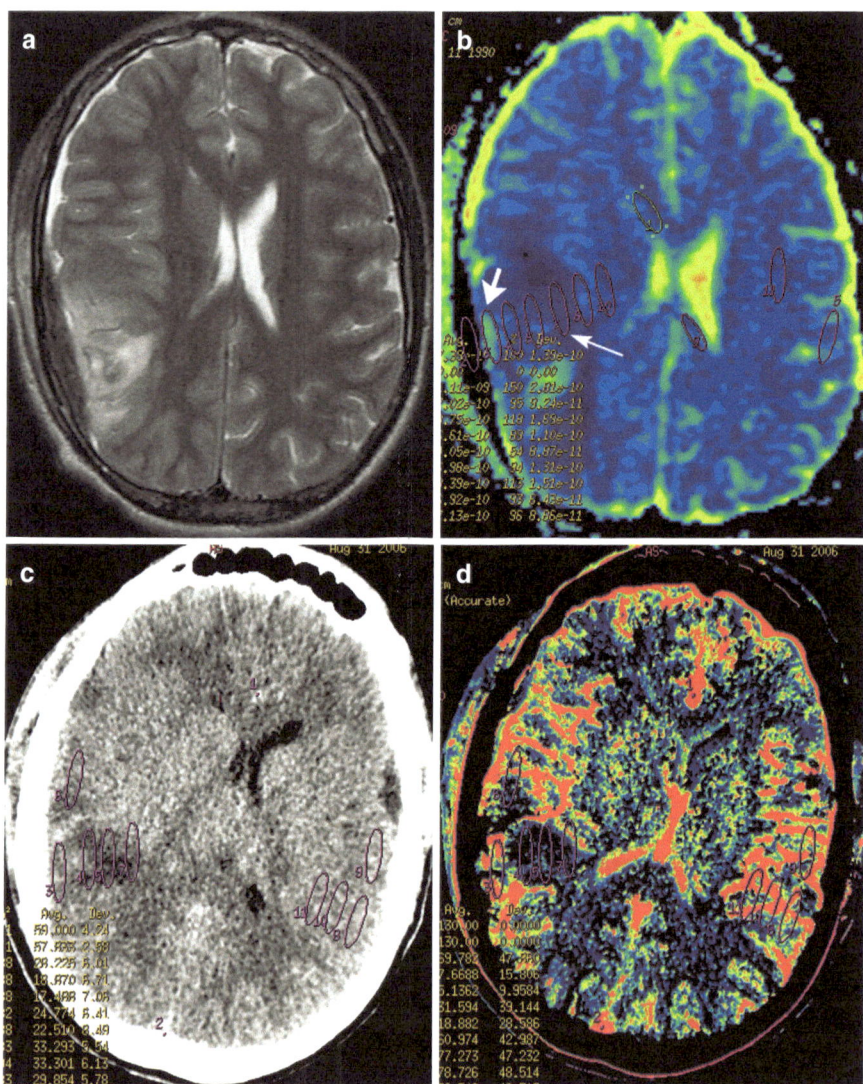

Fig. 6.4 Focal contusion and epidural hematoma in the right temporoparietal region. MRI in 5 days after trauma: T2WI (**a**); ADC map (**b**) shows combination of vasogenic (1.1×10^{-3} mm²/c, *short white arrow*) and cytotoxic (0.4×10^{-3} mm²/c, *long white arrow*) edema in the perifocal zone of focal contusion. CT and CT perfusion (**c, d**) in 5 days and 12 days (**e, f**) after trauma

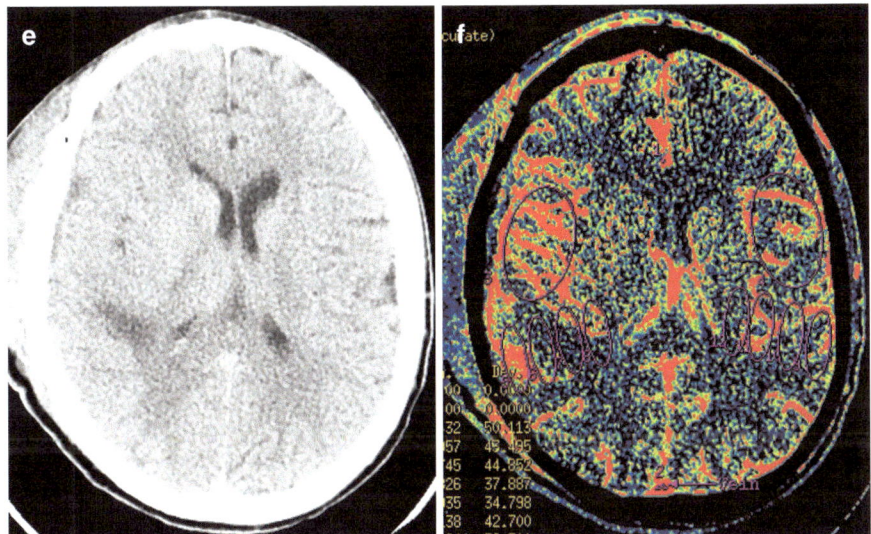

Fig. 6.4 (continued)

recovery of consciousness and preservation of the mild left-sided hemiparesis. Conventional CT after surgery showed an enlarged volume of the right hemisphere with low-density frontotemporal and basal ganglia areas. Perfusion CT studies in 3 and 9 days after injury demonstrated an rCBF elevation in the hemisphere on the removed hematoma site with the maximal ICP values not exceeding 20 mmHg (Fig. 6.7).

It is necessary to note that enlargement of the right hemisphere volume, according to perfusion CT studies, was caused by the increased rCBF in combination with brain edema. Diffusion-tensor MRI has also proved these data. MRI examinations showed that a combination of two pathophysiological phenomena –hyperemia and brain edema – in the acute period of trauma caused development of pathomorphological (cystic-atrophic) changes in the brain and persistent neurological symptoms (Fig. 6.8). EEG recordings (in 18 months after TBI) showed depression of the cortical activity in the right frontal lobe. These changes are typical for brain atrophy. Two-stage sharp evoked epileptiform potentials of theta wave prevailed on the left side, more in the temporo-fronto-central regions, thus suggesting the regions of irritation. These zones were located in the basal temporal (close to the midline) structures of the left hemisphere.

Similarly, the first and second MR tractography studies in this patient demonstrated corpus callosum fibers shortening in its different parts, more on the right. However, repeated MRI (in 7 months and 18 months) visualized some "lost" fibers, which cannot be explained only by decreased edema or improved diffusion along the axons (Fig. 6.9).

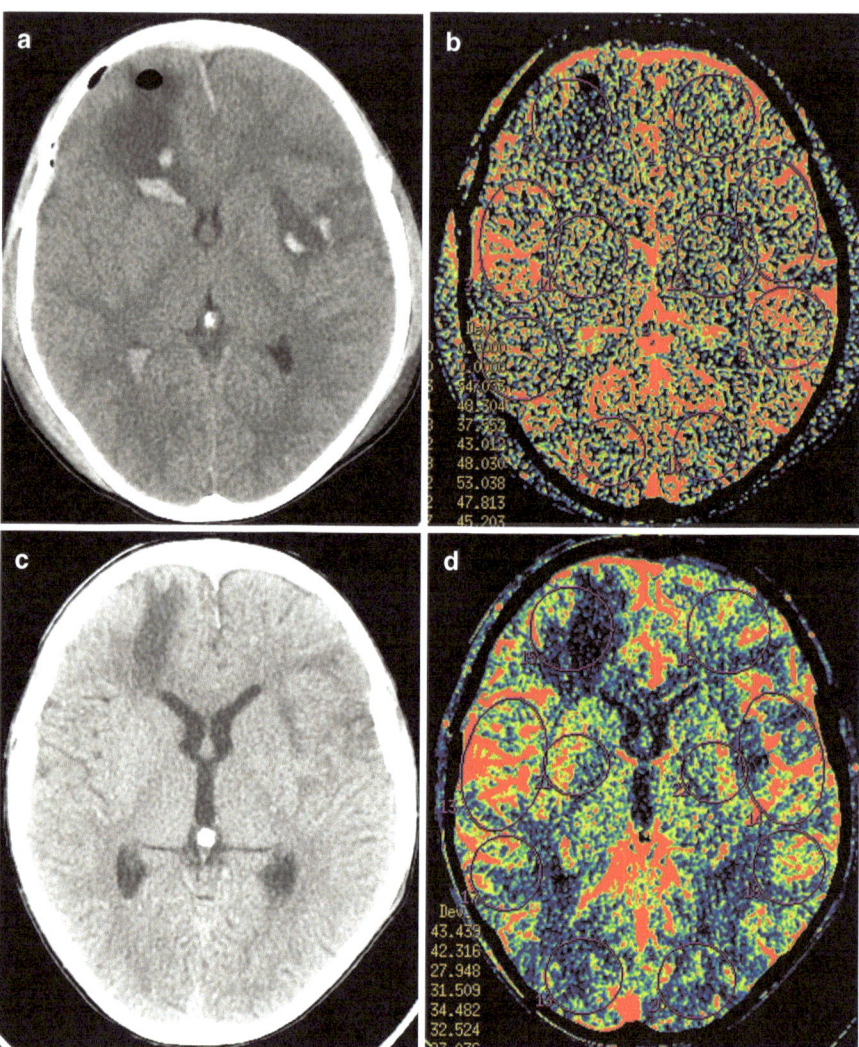

Fig. 6.5   M., 6 y.o. Severe TBI resulting from an object drop on the head. GCS, 8. Coma duration, 8 days. Outcome, moderate disability. CT and CT perfusion (**a, b**) in 3 days after trauma show hemorrhagic focal contusions in the right frontal and left frontotemporal regions, intraventricular hemorrhage, reduction of rCBF values in the right frontal lobe. CT and CT perfusion (**c, d**) in 12 days reveal decrease of perifocal edema, further rCBF reduction in the right frontal lobe, appearance of rCBF reduction zones in the left frontotemporal region. MRI study (T2WI, **e, f**) in 3 years after trauma demonstrates cystic-atrophic areas, which correspond to the reduction of rCBF value areas in CT perfusion studies

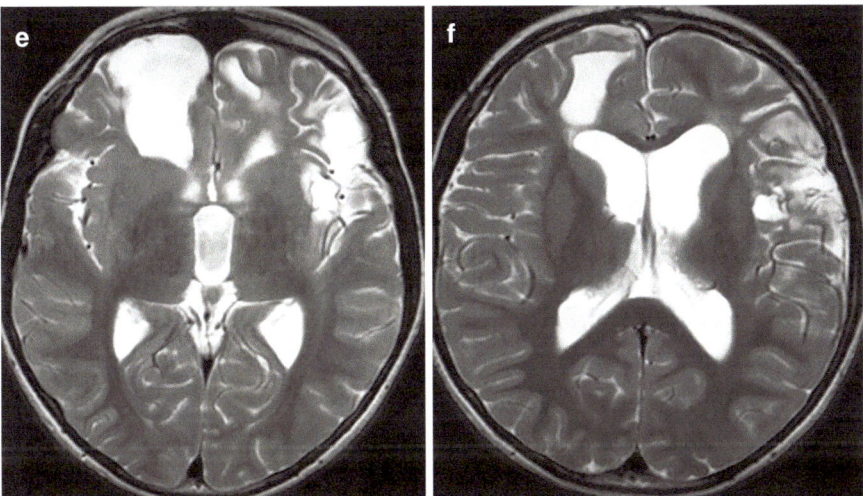

Fig. 6.5 (continued)

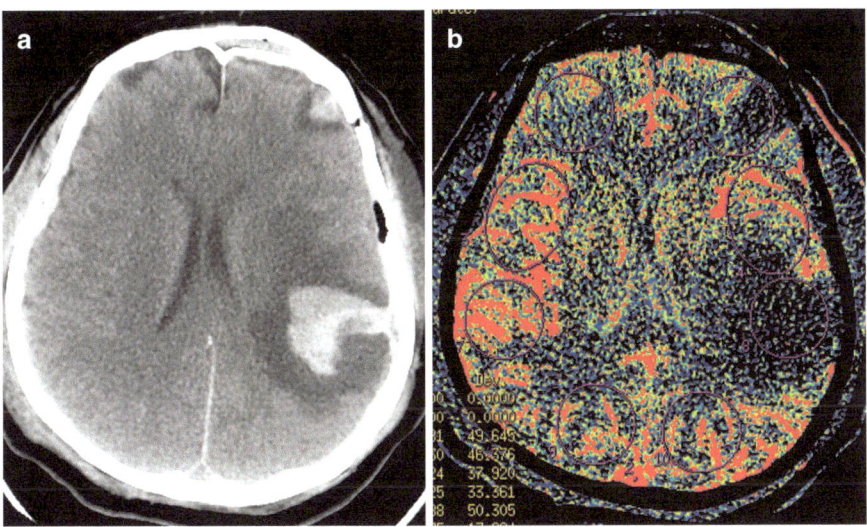

Fig. 6.6 Dynamic CT and CT perfusion data in a 49 y.o. patient after removal of a subdural hematoma in the left frontoparietotemporal region; (**a**, **b**) 4 days after trauma and after hematoma removal, coma, GCS (7), (**c**, **d**) 13 days after trauma, emerging from coma (*see explanation in the text*)

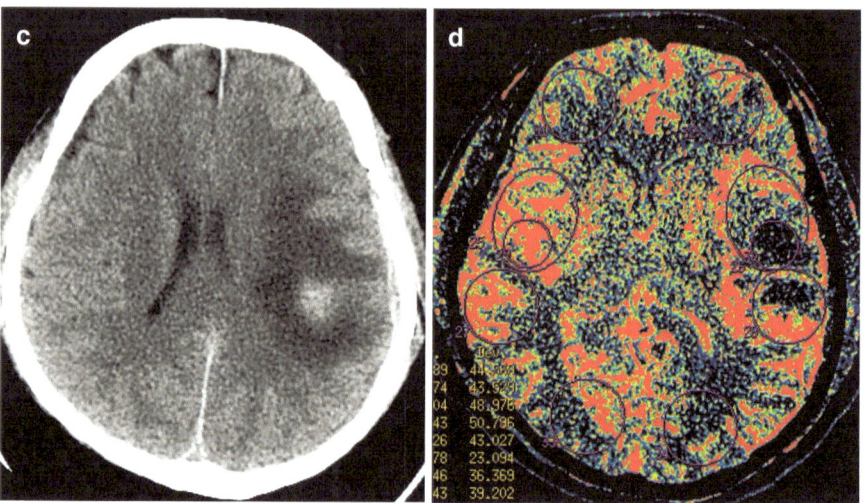

Fig.6.6 (continued)

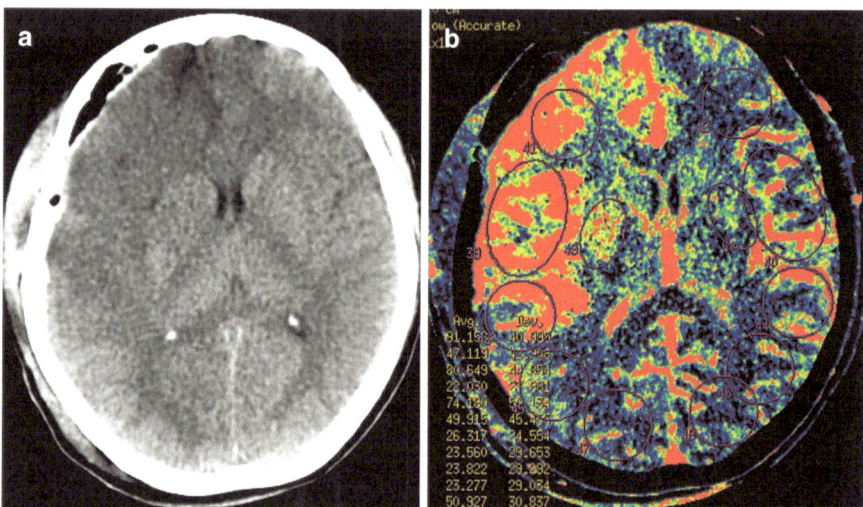

Fig. 6.7 F., 17 y.o. Traffic accident. GCS, 7. Outcome, moderate disability. CT and MRI studies after removal of subdural hematoma of the right frontotemporal region. CT perfusion in 3 days (**a**, **b**) and 9 days (**d**, **e**) after injury reveals persistent hyperemia in the right ACA and MCA vascular regions; DWI MRI (**c**) (in 3 days after injury) reveals signs of cytotoxic edema corresponding to the hyperemia zone (*red color* on rCBF maps)

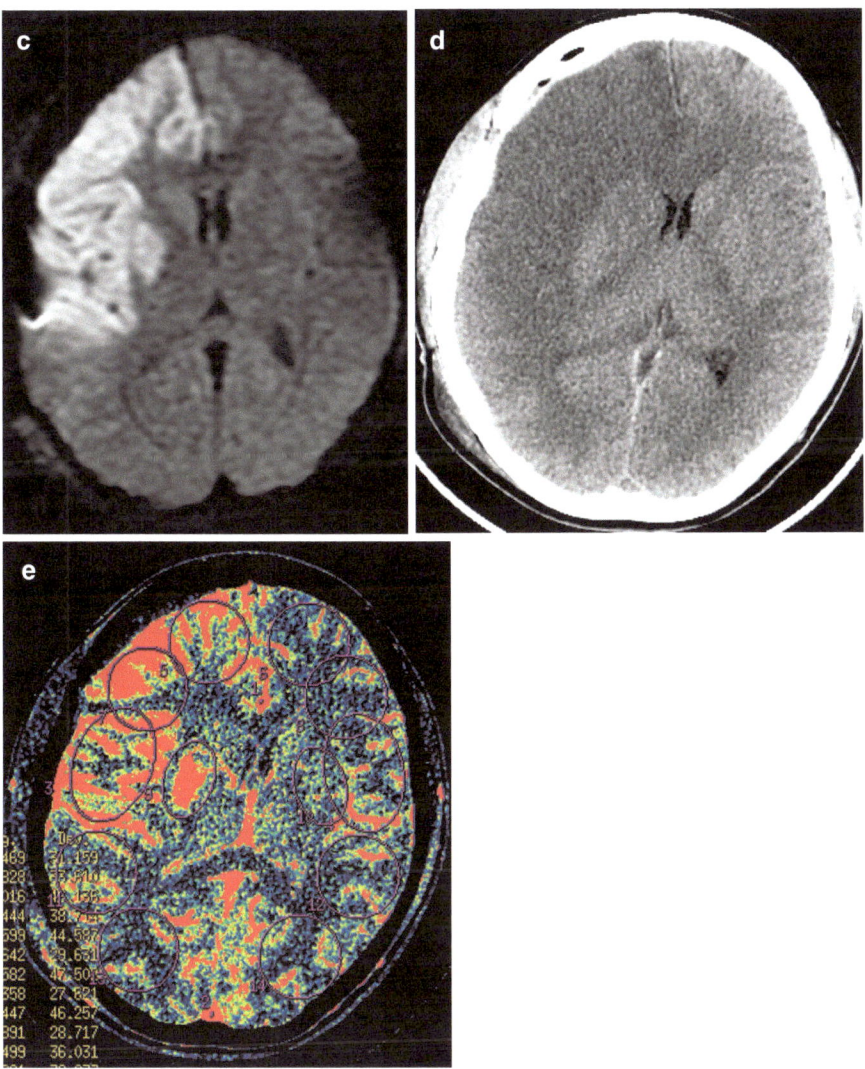

Fig. 6.7 (continued)

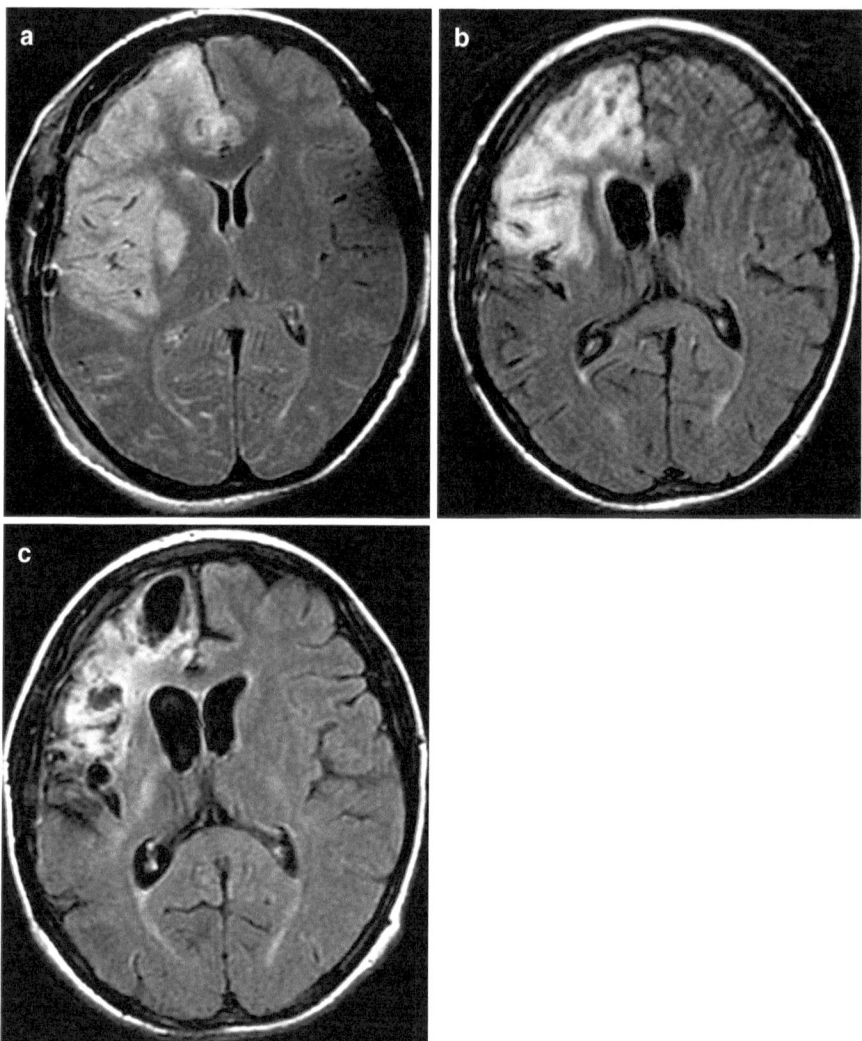

Fig. 6.8 MRI dynamics (see Fig. 6.7). T2-FLAIR in 3 days after injury (**a**), in 1.5 months (**b**), and 7 months (**c**) reveals cystic-atrophic changes in the right frontal and temporal lobes

6.3   Analysis of rCBF in the Brain Stem

Cerebral blood flow was evaluated in 24 patients both in hemispheric and brain stem structures at the midbrain level: 4 patients had mild TBI (GCS of 13–15) and 20 were in coma (GCS ≤ 8). Brain stem blood flow parameters in patients with mild TBI ranged 17.1–38.6 ml/100 g/min (average 25.2 ± 7). In 7 of 20 patients in coma

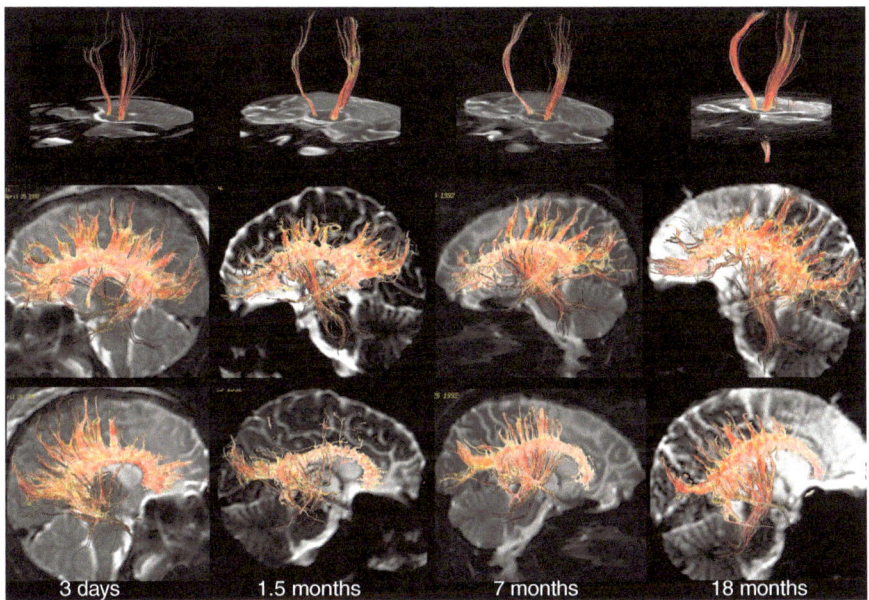

Fig. 6.9 Dynamic MR tractography in a patient with severe TBI (see Figs. 6.7 and 6.8) after removal of the right-sided subdural hematoma. Changes of the corticospinal tracts (*upper row*) and corpus callosum (left view, *middle row*; right view, *lower row*) in different periods after trauma (3 days; 1.5, 7, 18 months)

on admission with subsequent favorable outcome, rCBF values ranged 18.5–51.4 ml/100 g/min (average 26.4 ± 8).

In 13 of 20 patients with unfavorable outcome, rCBF values ranged 4.0–42.9 ml/100 g/min (average 27.6 ± 7). In 3 of them with primary brain stem damage (Fig. 6.10), the blood flow in the injured brain stem was ranged 4.0–12.2 ml/100 g/min. The other patient had secondary brain stem damage with brain stem blood flow parameters ranged 3.6–9.2 ml/100 g/min (Fig. 6.11).

Low value of the brain stem blood flow (12.2 ml/100 g/min) was revealed in hemorrhagic focus in the right thalamus and right cerebral peduncle in DAI patient in coma (GCS of 5). Blood flow value in the left cerebral peduncle was 30.1 ml/100 g/min (Fig. 6.12). Later on, this patient emerged from coma, however, retained neurological signs of a deep persistent left-sided hemiparesis. Dynamic MRI in 33 and 77 days following injury showed a cyst formation in the right cerebral peduncle (in the zone of hemorrhage and reduced blood flow). MR tractography detected increasing thinning of the right corticospinal tract (see Figs. 4.14 and 4.15, Chap. 4).

According to our data analysis, brain stem blood flow values in patients with mild TBI had a more narrow range (18.0–38.0 ml/100 g/min) compared to analogous parameters in patients in coma, especially followed by unfavorable outcome (Fig. 6.13).

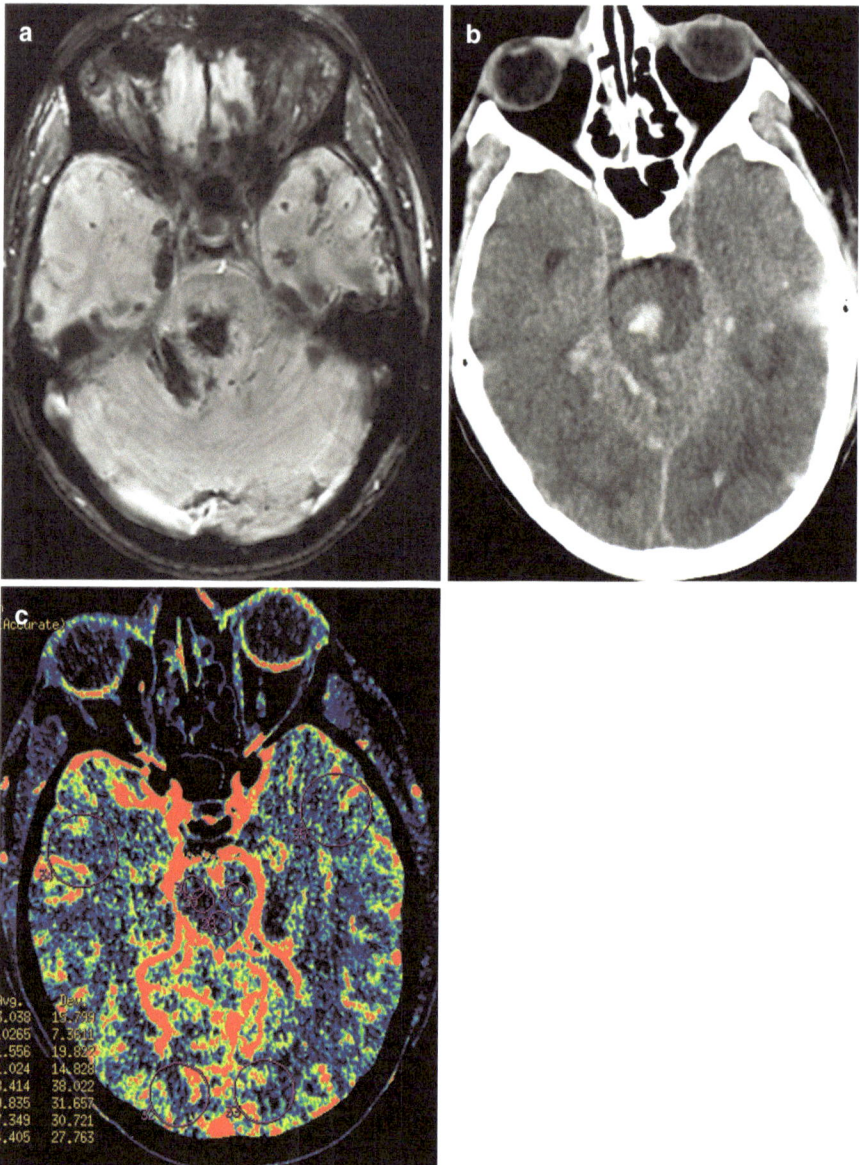

Fig. 6.10 M., 30 y.o. Traffic accident. Diffuse axonal injury with a primary brain stem damage. GCS, 4. Outcome, severe disability (minimally conscious state, tetraparesis). SWAN modality of MRI (**a**) and CT (**b**) show hemorrhagic lesions in the brain stem, temporal lobes, and cerebellar hemispheres. Blood flow values on map (**c**) in the right and middle parts of the midbrain – 4.0– 12.2 ml/100 g/min

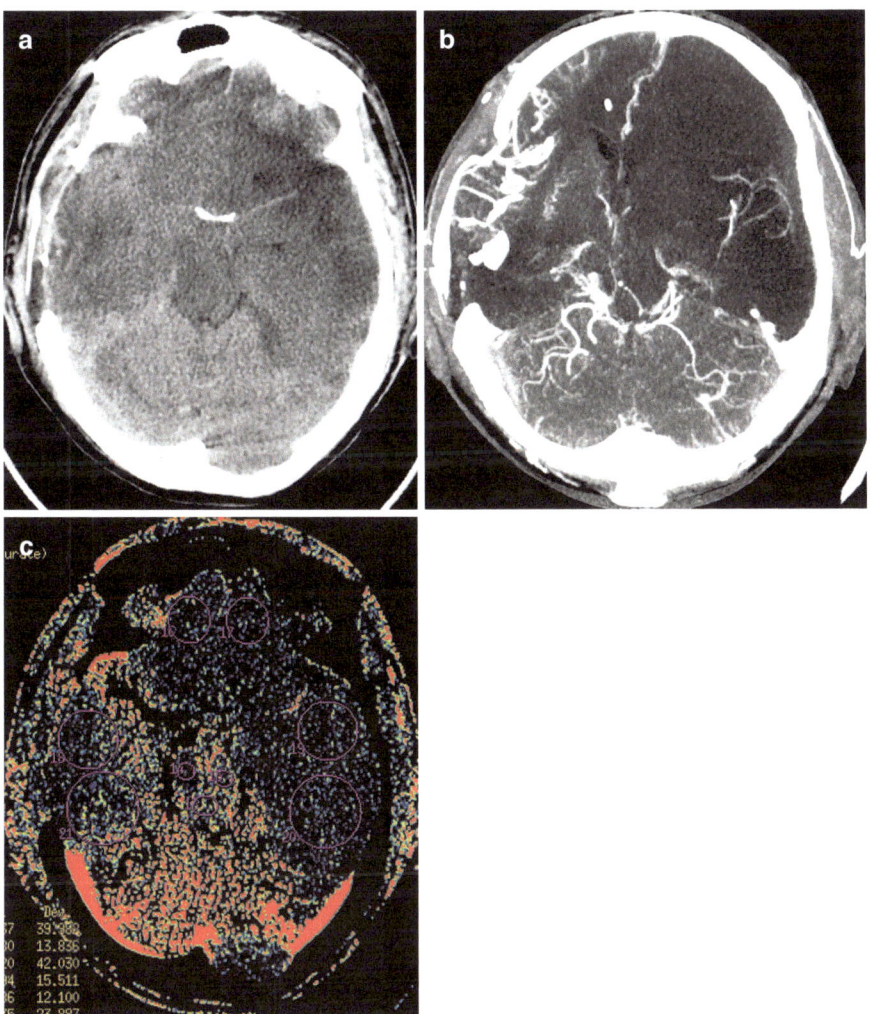

Fig. 6.11 M., 36 y.o. Gunshot injury. Penetrating craniocerebral injury. CT (**a**), CT angiography (**b**), and CT perfusion (**c**) in 16 days after injury and right-sided craniectomy. Transtentorial herniation, secondary ischemia; GCS, 3. Blood flow values are decreased in the right part of the midbrain (3.6 ml/100 g/min), in the frontal and temporal lobes (3.0–4.2 ml/100 g/min)

6.4 Dynamic Studies of rCBF in the Brain Stem

Dynamic rCBF studies at the midbrain level were conducted in 18 patients in coma; 8 of them had favorable and 10 unfavorable outcome.

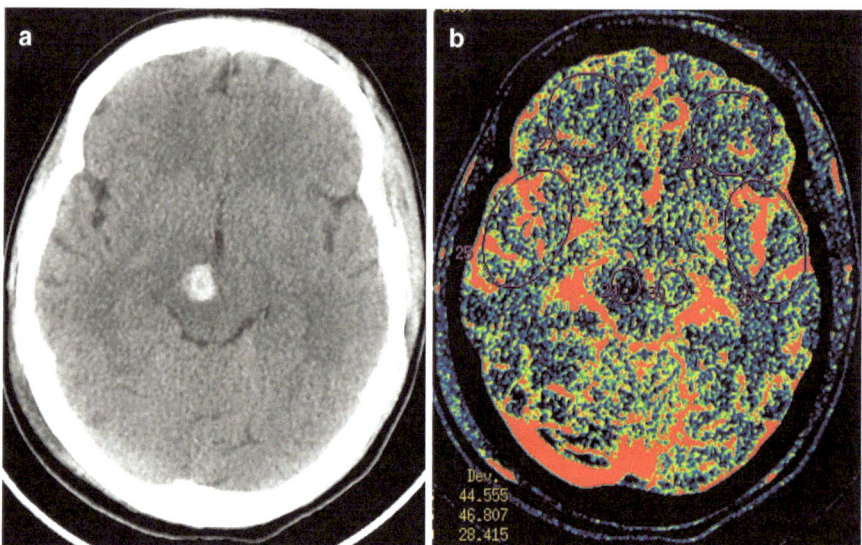

Fig. 6.12 Traffic accident. Severe TBI; GCS, 5. 4 days after injury (CT, **a**; CT perfusion, **b**). Left-sided hemiparesis in 6 months after trauma (*see explanation in the text*)

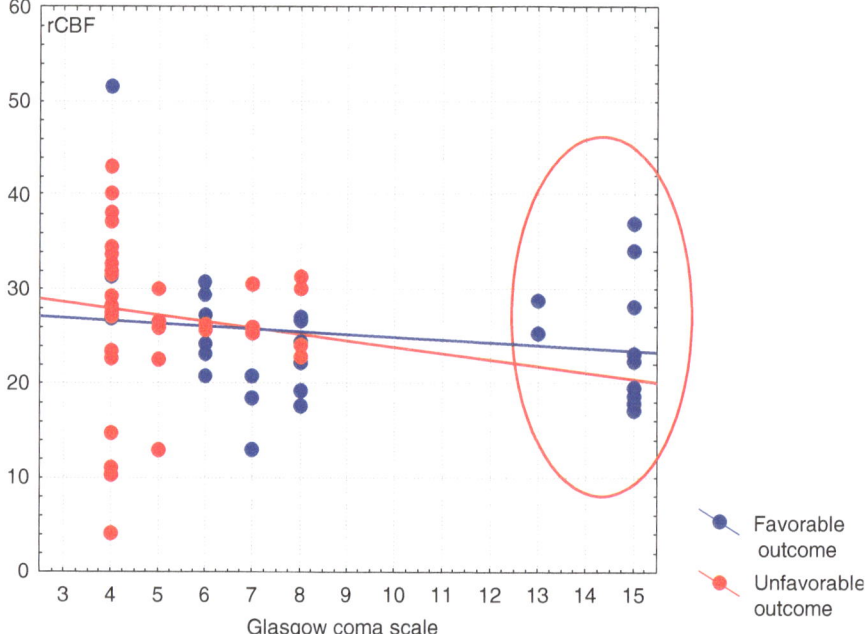

Fig. 6.13 Average rCBF values in the brain stem in comatose patients with favorable (*n* = 7, *blue*) and unfavorable outcomes (*n* = 13, *red*) and patients with mild TBI in a conscious state (*n* = 4, *red oval*)

CT perfusion study in eight patients in coma and with subsequent favorable outcome showed brain stem blood values ranging 18.5–42.9 ml/100 g/min in 1–5 days following injury. After emergence from coma, dynamic CT perfusion within 8–27 days following trauma demonstrated the blood flow range of 18.6–49.6 ml/100 g/min. The average rCBF values in hemispheric and brain stem structures in eight patients in coma and with subsequent favorable outcome obtained by initial CT perfusion did not significantly differ from those with repeated CT perfusion studies (Fig. 6.14).

CT perfusion studies in 10 patients with unfavorable outcome performed within 1–9 days following injury revealed a wider range of blood flow values in the brain stem compared to patients with favorable outcome. However, average rCBF values did not differ significantly.

The most significant rCBF alterations in different vascular regions were revealed in 3 patients with severe injury and unfavorable outcome. In one of these patients (Fig. 6.15) with severe head injury, a comatose state was developed after a lucid interval as a result of brain dislocation increase. For these reasons, in the primary hospital, the patient underwent an immediate small craniectomy in the left temporoparietal region with a subdural hematoma removal. The next day the patient was transferred to the Burdenko Neurosurgery Institute. He was in deep coma (GCS, 4) at admission. CT scans showed extensive low-density areas in the left hemisphere and right frontal lobe, massive SAH, a right-sided 11-mm midline shift, and compression and deformation of basal cisterns accompanied by a small-sized bone defect in the left temporal area. A catheter was installed in the anterior horn of the right lateral ventricle for the measurement of ICP and CSF drainage. ICP was 60 mmHg, so the left-sided decompressive craniectomy was performed. Control CT studies visualized severe brain pathology described above. Perfusion CT studies demonstrated reduced rCBF values in the anterior cerebral arteries, left middle cerebral artery, and left posterior cerebral artery regions. The first (3 days after TBI) and repeated conventional CT and CT perfusion (5 days after TBI) examinations showed an extensive hemispheric edema and rCBF values ranging 18.5–49.6 ml/100 g/min in the cerebral peduncles. A wide-spectrum intensive therapy including hypothermia was undertaken; however, the patient died on the 8th day after TBI due to increased intracranial hypertension and brain herniation.

In the other case, a patient aged 47 sustained the combined trauma in a car accident. He had signs of DAI, hemorrhagic cerebellum contusion, intraventricular and subarachnoid hemorrhages, and occlusive hydrocephalus (Fig. 6.16a–c). On the 6th day, the patient's condition gradually deteriorated to a deep coma (GCS, 4) alongside with extracranial complications and increased intracranial hypertension (ICP > 30 mmHg). Routine CT and perfusion CT studies (Fig. 6.16d–f) demonstrated signs of diffuse edema and ischemia in both left and right territories of MCAs and PCAs (rCBF, 9.5 and 17.2 ml/100 g/min, correspondingly). Nevertheless, blood flow parameters at the cerebral peduncle level remained normal 32.8–34.4 ml/100 g/min. A deep coma was accompanied by development of bilateral mydriasis and disappearance of brain stem reflexes in 17 days after injury. The area of ischemia spread into vascular regions of both middle cerebral arteries and

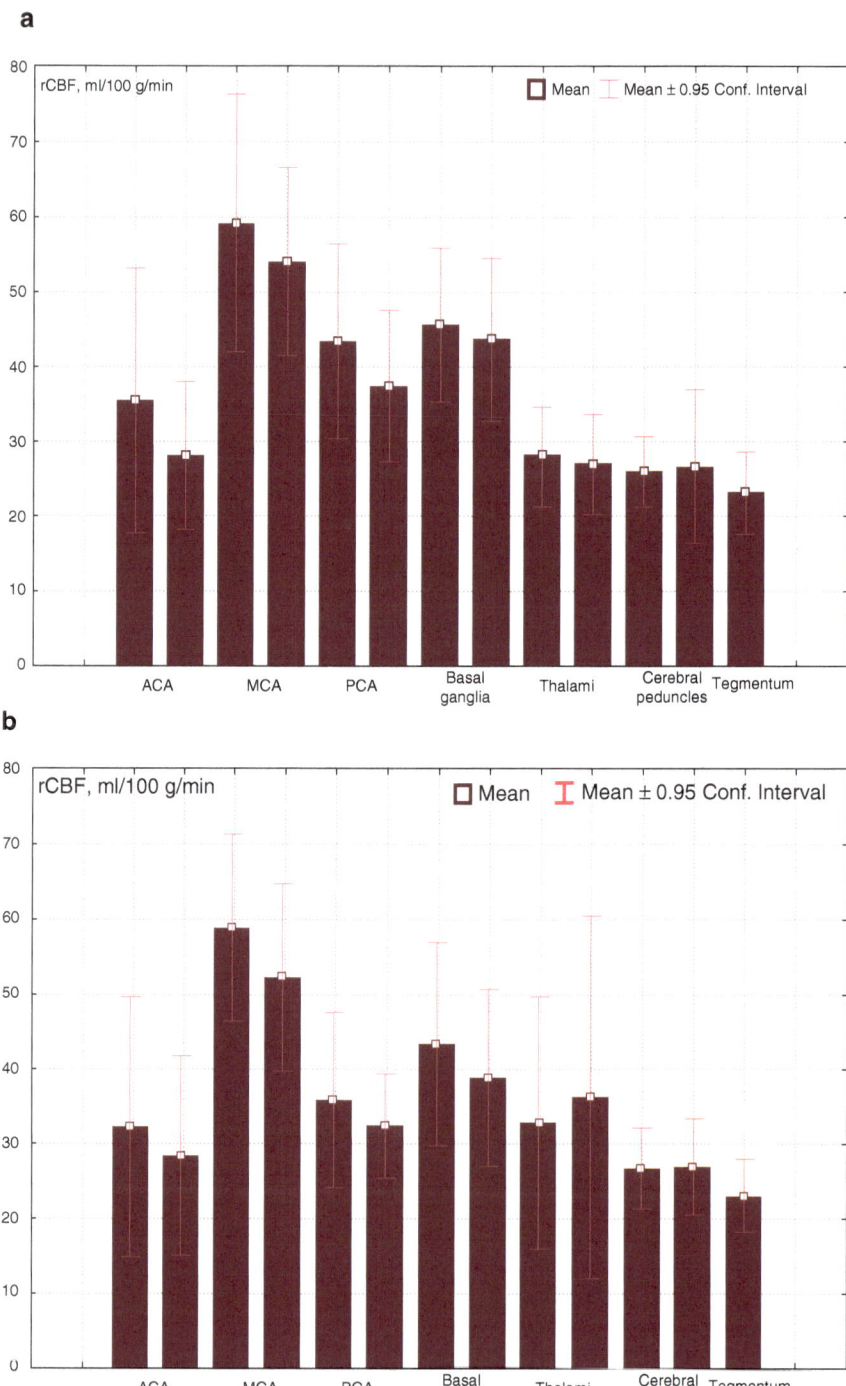

Fig. 6.14 Dynamics of average rCBF values in hemispheric and brain stem structures in 8 patients in coma with favorable outcome: (**a**) first study in 1–7 days; (**b**) second study in 8–30 days

terminal and central branches of PCA with brain stem involvement (Figs. 6.16g–i and 6.17). Blood flow values at the level of the cerebral peduncles were between 9.2 and 14.5 ml/100 g/min. CT angiography showed blood flow only in several branches of the middle cerebral arteries, anterior cerebral arteries, and superior and posterior inferior cerebellar arteries.

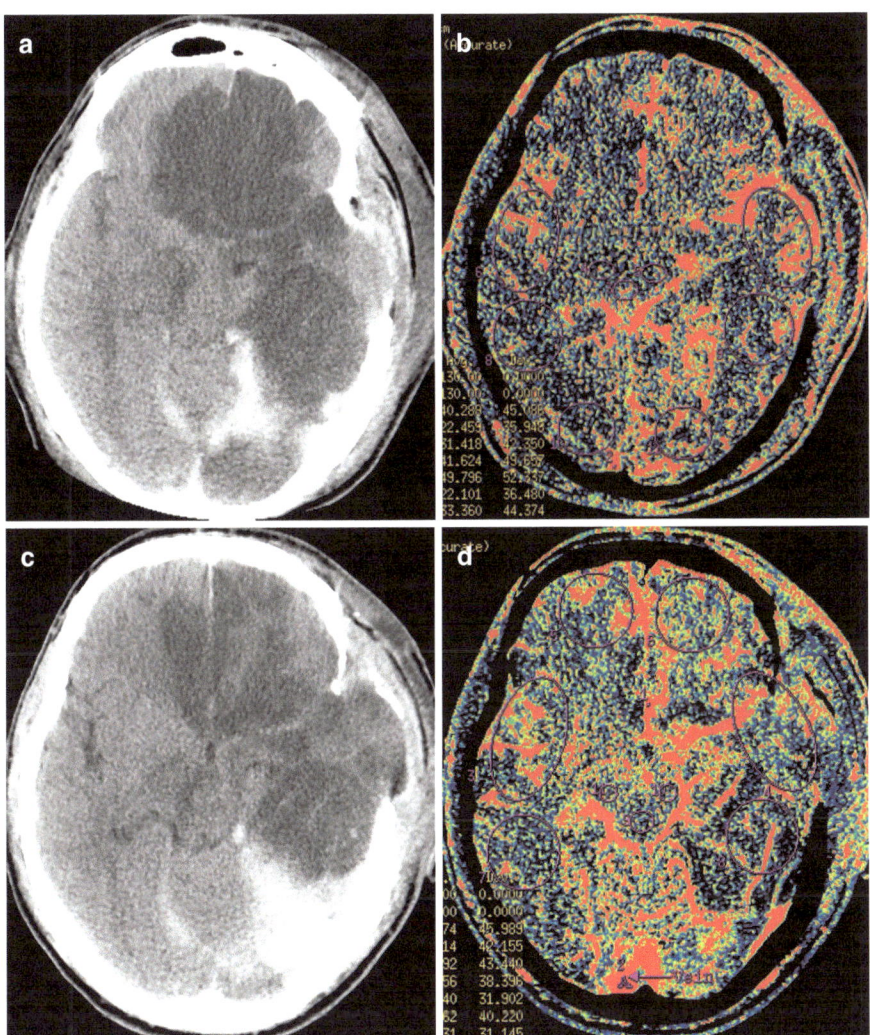

Fig. 6.15 M., 27 y.o. Focal contusions of the frontal and temporal lobes, secondary ischemia and edema in the left frontotemporal region and right frontal lobe. GCS, 4. Death in 8 days after injury and removal of the left-sided subdural hematoma. CT and rCBF map in 3 days (**a**, **b**); 5 days after trauma (**c**, **d**), uncontrolled intracranial hypertension ICP>60 mmHg. T2WI MRI in 8 days (**e**), transtentorial herniation signs; (**f**) MR angiography: absence of intracranial arteries visualization, MR signs of brain death

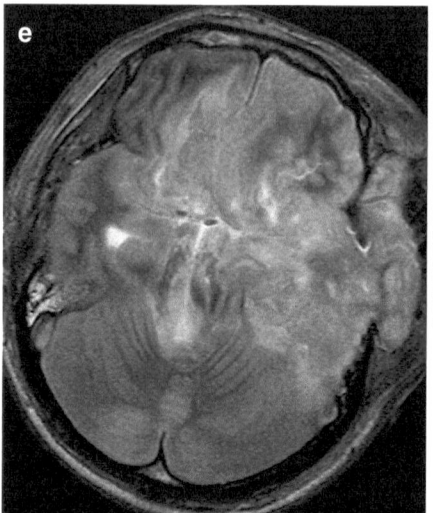
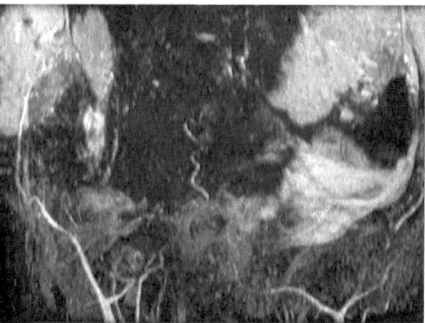

Fig. 6.15 (continued)

Separate analysis of cases with favorable and unfavorable outcome revealed a significant correlation between brain stem blood flow values and GCS in patients with favorable outcome ($p < 0.05$). Neither first nor second CT perfusion studies revealed such a significant correlation for patients with unfavorable outcome because they had variable (high and low) rCBF parameters (Figs. 6.18 and 6.19).

In our study, the regions of interest for brain stem blood flow measurements were standardized and included the midbrain parenchyma only. It explained the range of obtained blood flow values in the brain stem of patients in coma (both with favorable or unfavorable outcome). The data obtained suggest that blood flow in the brain stem, the most phylogenetically old brain structure, should have a resistant system of autoregulation. The lowest blood flow value (< 15 ml/100 g/min) in patients with primary or secondary brain stem damage might be regarded as the critical level.

6.5   Discussion

A wide application of modern neuroimaging technologies in diagnosis of TBI has fundamentally changed the algorithm of TBI management. Earlier X-ray studies were based on the descriptive anatomy of lesions only, considering neither

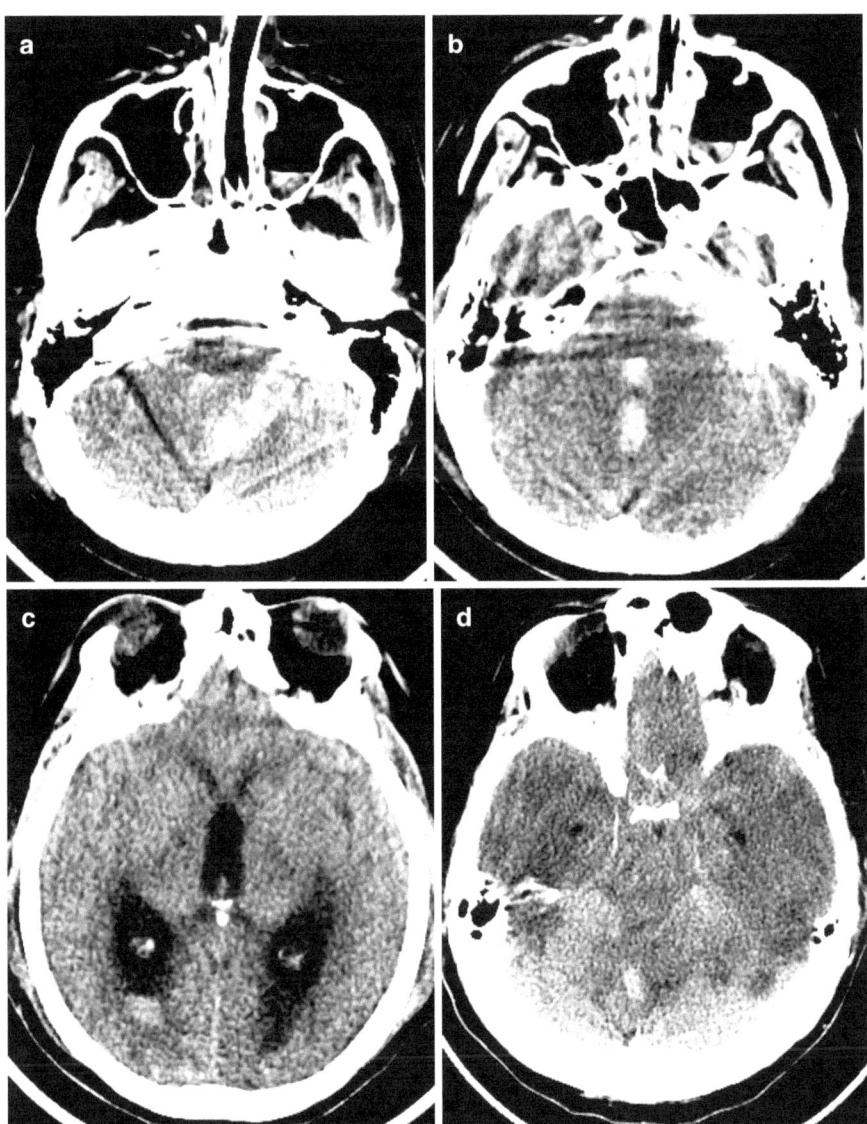

Fig. 6.16 M., 47 y.o. Severe combined TBI in a traffic accident. Diffuse axonal injury, hemorrhagic contusion in the left hemisphere and vermis of the cerebellum, subarachnoid and intraventricular hemorrhages. CT dynamics in 3 (**a–c**), 15 (**d–f**), and 17 (**g–i**) days after trauma. Regional rCBF maps (**c**, **f**, **i**) and CT angiography (**g**, **h**) demonstrate increasing ischemia in the brain stem, bilateral basal ganglia, and thalami

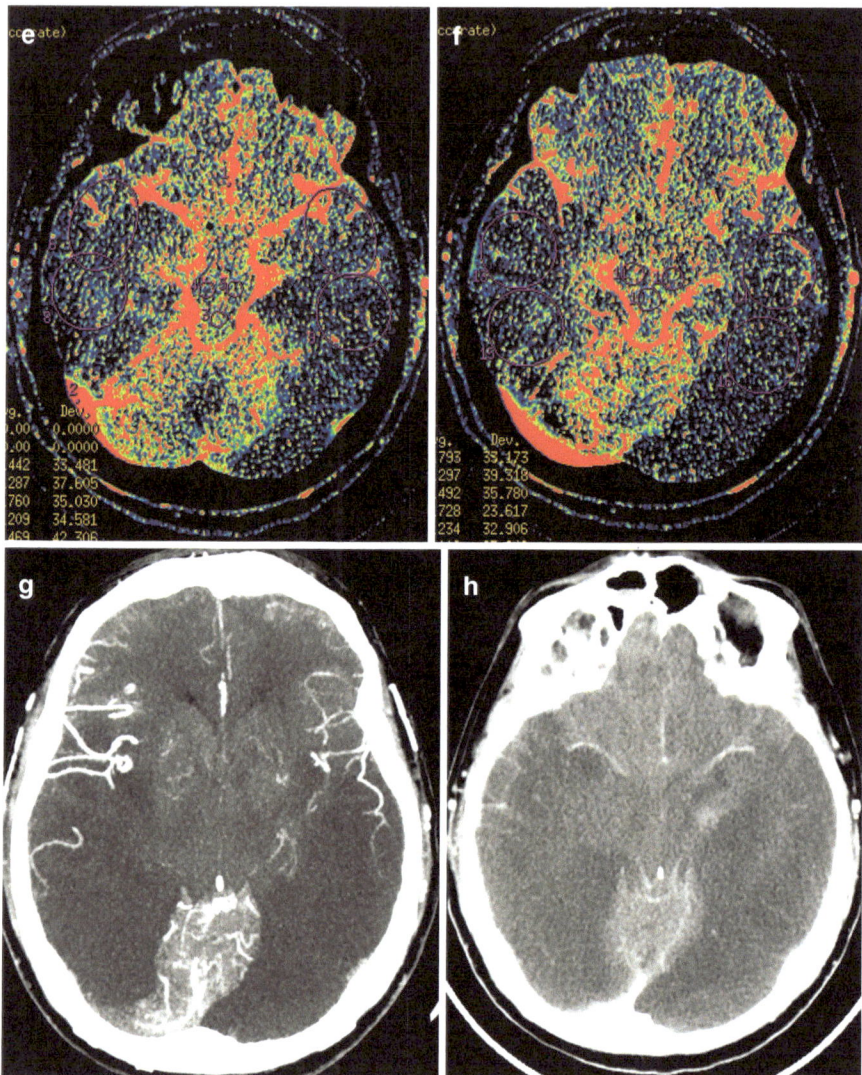

Fig. 6.16 (continued)

Fig.6.16 (continued)

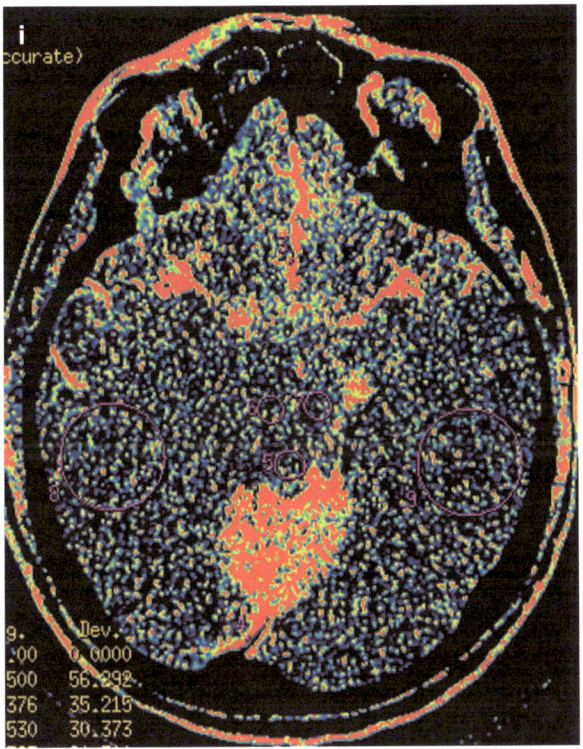

pathogenesis nor clinical manifestations or outcome of brain trauma. Recent advances in neuroimaging based on the fusion of anatomical and functional images have opened up new possibilities for understanding clinical symptoms, pathogenesis of the traumatic brain disease, and prognosis of outcome. New methods of neuroimaging allow exploring delicate pathophysiological and hemodynamic changes in the brain with their subsequent mapping. Perfusion CT study is a relatively modern method of CBF mapping which provides a quantitative evaluation of the regional cerebral blood flow (rCBF), cerebral blood volume (rCBV) values, and mean transit time (MTT) in patients with brain pathology. An evident correlation was demonstrated between the quantitative CT perfusion parameters and parameters obtained by other classical clinical methods of blood flow investigation (Wintermark et al. 2004). Earlier CT perfusion studies revealed peculiar rCBF alterations in hemispheric brain structures and main vascular regions in the acute phase after TBI (Wintermark et al. 2004; Zakharova et al. 2006; Soustiel et al. 2008).

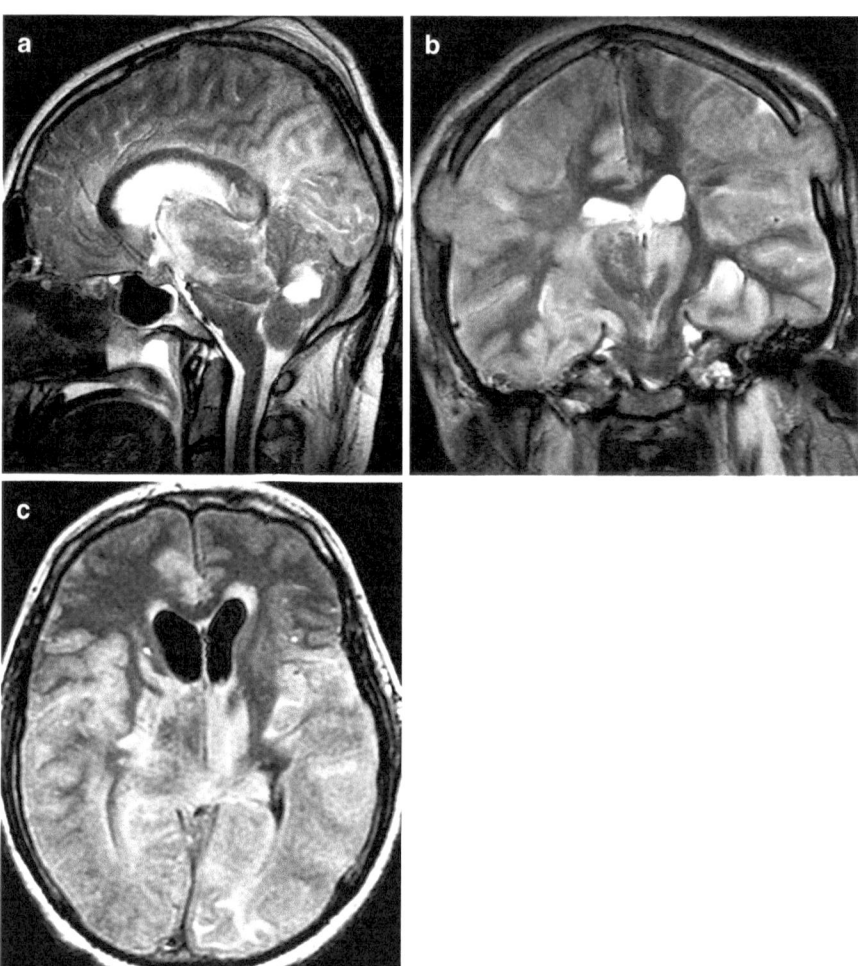

Fig. 6.17 (continuation of Fig. 6.16). Descending transtentorial herniation and secondary isch-emia developed within 15 days after injury; GCS, 3. Sagittal (**a**) and coronal (**b**) T2WI MRI reveal transtentorial herniation. T2-FLAIR (**c**) demonstrates bilateral zones of pathological MR signal increase

In this work for the first time, CT perfusion was used to evaluate the regional cerebral blood flow with regard to focal and diffuse morphological changes of the brain in severe trauma. Perfusion CT examinations were performed during the first week in the majority of patients and repeated in 2–4 weeks after TBI. Additional CT perfusion studies in 4–7 months following TBI were undertaken in two patients who developed hydrocephalus and were severely disabled.

Our studies showed that mosaic and multidirectional alterations of the cerebral blood flow may range from oligemia-ischemia in one vascular region to hyperemia

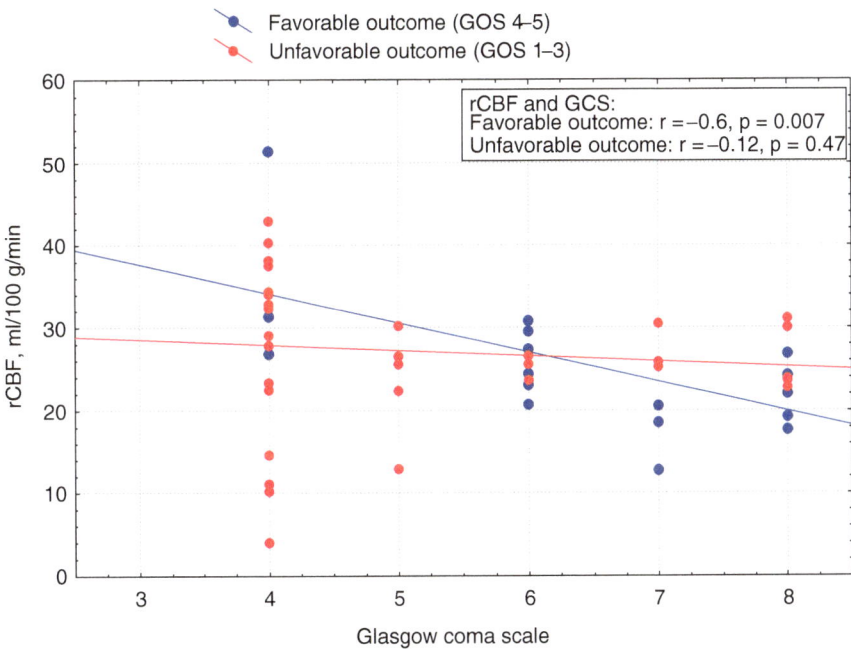

Fig. 6.18 Regional blood flow in the brain stem in comatose patients with favorable ($n = 8$) and unfavorable ($n = 10$) outcome, the first CT perfusion study in 1–7 days after trauma

in the other in dynamics of the traumatic brain disease. All patients in the analyzed group showed rCBF values beyond the normal range in the first and repeated CT perfusion examinations.

The lowest rCBF values in hemispheric structures were identified in hemorrhagic contusions within the first 3 days after injury (16.9 ± 6.0 ml/100 g/min), with a tendency to decrease in the following days. Dynamic CT and MRI studies showed that hemorrhagic contusions of cortical-subcortical localization with a marked rCBF reduction usually resulted in focal cystic-atrophic changes of brain tissues.

Based on dynamic CT and MRI data, we have shown for the first time that persistent regional "luxury" hyperperfusion combined with edema may lead to severe atrophic changes of the brain, so typical for contusions and ischemia.

Resistant regional ischemia in some of our patients, regardless of maintenance of cerebral perfusion pressure, may be due to primary traumatic damage of the brain tissues and vessels or be the result of a secondary vascular response to parenchymatous and subarachnoid hemorrhage, brain compression by hematoma, venous outflow disturbance, and sludge syndrome. At the same time, in some patients CT perfusion showed normalization of rCBF parameters in the contusion area in dynamics. In cases when rCBF values could not reach their physiological range and persistent ischemia or hyperemia was present, the brain tissue atrophic transformation developed.

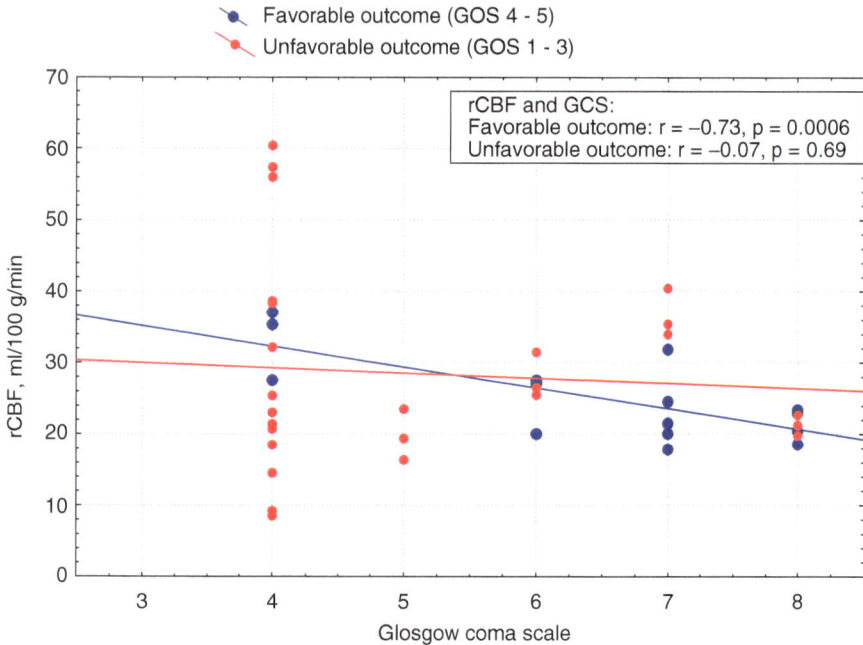

Fig. 6.19 Regional blood flow in the brain stem in comatose patients with favorable ($n=8$) and unfavorable ($n=10$) outcome, the second CT perfusion study in 8–30 days after trauma

The problem of critical rCBF levels in different brain structures following traumatic injury has long been recognized. However, each of the modern clinical neuroimaging methods requires its own correction and interpretation. Having compared xenon-enhanced CT and perfusion CT data, the identical rCBF average values with inclusion (70.0 ± 14.0 ml/100 g/min) or exclusion of large cerebral artery branches (42.0 ± 26.0 ml/100 g/min) were obtained. Average rCBF values were separately obtained for the gray matter (68.0 ± 13.0 ml/100 g/min) and white matter (26.0 ± 10.0 ml/100 g/min) as well as for pathological brain tissues (14.0 ± 10.0 ml/100 g/min) (Wintermark et al. 2001). Analogous low rCBF values in hemispheric hemorrhagic focal contusions were obtained by perfusion CT in the research of Soustiel et al. (2008) and in our earlier series of patients (Zakharova et al. 2006, 2012; Zakharova 2013; Potapov et al. 2011).

At the same time, there is no information in the literature about CT perfusion data on dynamic blood flow changes in the brain stem of patients in coma and during consciousness recovery (or non-recovery). It was determined in this work that average blood flow values in the brain stem in comatose patients with different outcome and in different periods of consciousness recovery were similar to the analogous values in patients with less severe trauma and in states of moderate obnubilation or clear consciousness (GCS 13–15). The lowest rCBF values (3.6–9.2 ml/100 g/min) in the brain stem were detected in 3 patients with primary hemorrhagic damages and in a patient with signs of brain stem compression with further death. These data suggest that blood flow in the brain stem has strong mechanisms of autoregulation. An increase of the arterial pressure is considered as one of the universal mechanisms for maintaining constant blood flow values in the brain stem (Cushing's reflex) as a response to ischemia. This hypothesis was supported by experimental studies of Zierski et al. (1983) and Nagao et al. (1984). It was shown that an increase of ICP resulted in a decrease of rCBF in supratentorial structures (including the basal ganglia and thalami) earlier than in the brain stem. Besides, the blood flow values for the thalamus (37.5 ml/100 g/min), inferior colliculus (42.1 ml/100 g/min), and medulla oblongata (30.7 ml/100 g/min) have been established (Nagao et al. 1984). Noradrenergic structure of the reticular formation, presented by the nucleus locus coeruleus, might be responsible for realization of Cushing's reflex. It is well known that this structure has also a modulating effect on the global cortex activity (Clark et al. 1987; Parvizi and Damasio 2003). In our studies, blood flow values in the hemorrhagic brain stem damage areas and supratentorial focal contusions of the mixed density were similar to those obtained by CT perfusion in a study by Soustiel et al. (2008) in the hemorrhagic foci and to those in the zones of ischemia obtained by xenon-enhanced CT and CT perfusion methods (Wintermark et al. 2001). At the same time, xenon-enhanced CT studies (Ritter et al. 1999) in a series of patients with severe brain injury revealed a significantly wider range of blood flow values at the midbrain level. For all that, significantly worse outcomes were marked when rCBF values were ≤40.0 ml/100 g/min, and in 1 year 8 of 9 patients with the brain blood flow below 20.0 ml/100 g/min were dead, and the other was severely disabled. Such a great difference in rCBF values in the brain stem obtained by xenon-enhanced CT studies of patients in coma might be explained by including the whole midbrain section (with branches or basilar artery main trunk, as well) into the region of interest. The regions of interest in our study included midbrain parenchyma only, thus explaining a more narrow, low range blood flow values in the brain stem in cases of coma (with favorable or unfavorable outcomes). Further studies will allow outlining predictive valuable blood flow values for the brain stem based on perfusion CT data.

References

Clark C, Geffen G, Geffen L (1987) Catecholamines and attention: animal and clinical studies. Neurosci Biobehav Rev 11:341–352

Nagao S, Sunami N, Tutsui T et al (1984) Acute intracranial hypertension and brain- stem blood flow. An experimental study. J Neurosurg 60(3):566–571

Parvizi J, Damasio A (2003) Neuroanatomical correlates of brainstem coma. Brain 126: 1524–1536

Potapov A, Zakharova N, Pronin I et al (2011) Prognostic value of ICP, CPP and regional blood flow monitoring in diffuse and focal traumatic cerebral lesions. Zh Vopr Neirokhir Im N N Burdenko 75(3):3–16

Pronin I, Fadeeva L, Zakharova N, Dolgushin M, Kornienko V (2007) Perfusion CT: evaluation of cerebral blood flow in normal subject. Med Visualiz 3:8–12

Ritter A, Muizelaar J, Barnes T et al (1999) Brain stem blood flow, papillary response, and outcome in patients with severe head injuries. Neurosurgery 44(5):941–948

Soustiel J, Mahamid E, Goldsher D, Zaaroor M (2008) Perfusion CT for early assessment of traumatic cerebral contusion. Neuroradiology 50:189–196

Wintermark M, Thiran JP, Maeder P et al (2001) Simultaneous measurements of regional cerebral blood flow by perfusion-CT and stable xenon-CT: a validation study. AJNR Am J Neuroradiol 22:905–914

Wintermark M, van Melle G, Schnyder P et al (2004) Admission perfusion CT: prognostic value in patients with severe head trauma. Radiology 232:211–220

Zakharova N (2013) Neuroimaging of structural and hemodynamic disturbances in severe traumatic brain injury (clinical CT – MRI studies). Dissertation, Burdenko Neurosurgery Institute, Moscow

Zakharova N, Potapov A, Pronin I et al (2006) Investigation of regional cerebral blood flow volume in patients with injuries and its consequences using CT-perfusion method. In: Abstracts of the European Society of Neuroradiology XXXI congress, Geneva, 13–16 Sept 2006. Neuroradiology 48(Suppl 2):164

Zakharova N, Potapov A, Kornienko V, Pronin I et al (2012) Perfusion CT study of brain stem blood flow in patients with traumatic brain injuries. In: Abstracts of 36th European Society of Neuroradiology annual meeting, Edinburgh, 19–23 Sept 2012. Neuroradiology 54(Suppl 1): 136

Zierski J, Kurzai E, Hoffman O et al (1983) Cerebral blood flow in the brainstem during increased ICP. In: Ishii S, Nagai H, Brock M (eds) Intracranial pressure. Springer, Berlin, pp 452–457

Index

A

Apparent diffusion coefficient (ADC), 31, 32
  contralateral to hemiparesis, 72, 73
  control group, 70–72
  corpus callosum, genu and splenium,
    73–75
  cytotoxic and vasogenic edema, 7
  homolateral to hemiparesis, 71–73
  patients without paresis, 71
  tetraparesis, 74
  water diffusion and anisotropy
    disturbances, 35
Arterial spin labeling method (ASL), 11, 12

B

Burdenko Neurosurgery Institute, 25, 69,
    85, 143

C

Cerebral blood flow (CBF)
  assessment
    arterial spin labeling method, 12
    CT perfusion method, 11, 13–14
    ICP monitoring, 13
    MR perfusion method, 12
    PET/SPECT, 11
    XeCT, 11
    xenon, 11
  clinical material
    clinical and instrumental
      studies, 109–111
    Glasgow Coma Scale, 107
    inefficient conservative treatment, 107
    intracranial hypertension, 107
    MCA, 108
    TBI severity, 108
  CT perfusion, 120
  intracranial hypertension, 122

long-term coma, 120
rCBF, patients
  combined DAI, 115–117
  contusion areas, 119
  diffuse axonal injury, 112–115
  focal brain contusions, 117–119
  regional hypoperfusion (oligemia)/
    ischemia, 121
Classification
  CT classification (*see* Computed
    tomography (CT))
  Firsching's classification, 42, 43, 50, 52
  Marshall's classification, 30
  MRI classification (*see* Magnetic
    resonance imaging (MRI))
Clinical and prognostic value
  cerebral blood flow assessment
    arterial spin labeling method, 12
    CT perfusion method, 11, 13–14
    ICP monitoring, 13
    MR perfusion method, 12
    PET/SPECT, 11
    XeCT, 11
    xenon, 11
  classifications, 4
  computed tomography, 5–6
  DT MRI
    anatomical structures, 9
    application, 10
    commissural and projection
      pathways, 11
    diffusion characteristics, 10
    immunocytochemical method, 10
    qualitative and quantitative
      assessment, 10
    structural degeneration, 11
  MRI
    classification of, 8
    DWI, 7
    1H MR spectroscopy, 7–8

N. Zakharova et al., *Neuroimaging of Traumatic Brain Injury*,
DOI 10.1007/978-3-319-04355-5, © Springer International Publishing Switzerland 2014

Clinical and prognostic value (*cont.*)
    susceptibility-weighted imaging, 6
    T2-FLAIR, 6
    T2* gradient echo sequences, 6
    T1-weighted imaging, 6
    T2-weighted imaging, 6
  neuroimaging methods, 8–9
  radiation safety, 14–16
  social and economic problems, 1–3
  structural and functional brain
    integrity, 3–4
Clinical evaluation
  clinical and morphological diagnosis, 28
  coma duration distribution, 27, 28
  computed tomography, 28–30
  Glasgow Outcome Scale, 26–28
  magnetic resonance tomography
    apparent diffusion coefficient, 31, 32
    corpus callosum, 31, 32
    corticospinal tracts, 31–33
    diffusion anisotropy, 31
    FA value, 31, 32
    two-dimensional color-coding
     maps, 31, 32
  patients aged distribution, 25, 26
  patients characteristics, 25–26
  statistical analysis, 33
  trauma mechanisms, 25, 26
Computed tomography (CT)
  clinical and prognostic value, 5–6
  vs. MRI, 61
    acute period of TBI, 35, 36
    corpus callosum damages, 35, 37, 39
    cortical-subcortical focal contusion,
     36, 42
    microhemorrhages, 36, 38, 43–46
    patient baseline characteristics, 35, 36
    posttraumatic cytotoxic edema, 36,
     39–41
    subacute subdural hematoma, 36, 42
    water diffusion and anisotropy
     disturbances, 35, 38–39
  regional cerebral blood flow
    average rCBF values, 143, 144, 152
    cerebral perfusion study, 126–128
    coma, decompressive craniectomy,
     129–131
    epidural hematoma, 129, 132–133
    focal contusion, 129, 132–133, 143,
     145–146
    gunshot injury, 139, 141
    increasing ischemia, 143, 147,
     149–150
    intracranial hypertension, 143, 147

    meningoencephalitis and
     hydrocephalus, 128–129
    persistent/increasing ischemia, 129,
     134–135
    primary brain stem damage, 139, 140
    subdural hematoma, 130, 133, 135–137
    xenon-enhanced CT study, 153
Corpus callosum and corticospinal tract
  dynamic DT-MRI study
    akinetic mutism, 101
    analyzed patients, characteristics
     of, 77–80
    atrophy, 84
    baldness of corpus callosum, 88
    brain pathways, 3D reconstructions
     of, 81
    brain structures, 89, 98
    CC and CST, 76
    coma, 97
    conductive pathways, 101
    craniotomy, 85
    DAI, acute stage of, 76
    density/shortening, fibers, 76, 82
    diffuse and focal brain damage, 86
    diffuse axonal injury, 75, 99
    DTI, 76
    fractional anisotropy, 92
    genu and splenium of CC, 97
    hemiparesis, 96
    MR tractography data, 85
    neurological disability, 86
    posttraumatic epilepsy
     and tetraparesis, 86
    pyramidal tract damage, 90
    spastic tetraparesis, 101
    T2-FLAIR, 92
    transient hemiparesis, 90
    vegetative state, 86
  quantitative DT-MRI analysis
    ADC and FA values, 70
    clinical outcome, 74
    contralateral to hemiparesis, 72
    cytotoxic edema, 73
    healthy volunteers, 70
    with hemiparesis, 73
    homolateral to hemiparesis, 72
    patients without paresis, 71
    with tetraparesis, 74
    vasogenic edema, 74
Corticospinal tracts (CST), 31–33
  CC and, 76, 99, 101, 102
  hemiparesis, 71, 72
  patients without paresis, 71
  tetraparesis, 74

Cranioplasty, 129–131
CT. *See* Computed tomography (CT)

D

DAI. *See* Diffuse axonal injury (DAI)
Decompressive craniectomy, 15, 30, 107, 117, 129, 130
Diffuse axonal injury (DAI), 9, 56, 82, 84, 86–88, 90
  acute stage, 76
  bilateral damages, midbrain level, 58
  coma, decompressive craniectomy, 130
  corpus callosum damage, 39
  and focal brain contusions, 92–93
  hemiparesis, 139, 142
  petechial hemorrhages, 43–46
  rCBF, 112–117
  severe DAI, 92
  subdural hematoma, 94
Diffusion-tensor imaging (DTI), 10, 11, 25, 35, 38–39, 76, 101
Diffusion-tensor MRI (DT MRI)
  clinical and prognostic value
    anatomical structures, 9
    application, 10
    commissural and projection pathways, 11
    diffusion characteristics, 10
    pathological processes, 10
    qualitative and quantitative assessment, 10
    structural degeneration, 11
  clinical evaluation
    apparent diffusion coefficient, 31, 32
    corpus callosum, 31, 32
    corticospinal tracts, 31–33
    FA value, 31, 32
    two-dimensional color-coding maps, 31, 32
Diffusion-weighted imaging (DWI), 7, 10, 12
  posttraumatic cytotoxic edema, 36, 39–41
  water diffusion and anisotropy disturbances, 35, 38–39

F

Fractional anisotropy (FA), 31, 32
  brain structures, 89
  changes of anisotropy, 35, 38–39
  contralateral to hemiparesis, 72
  control group, 70, 71
  corpus callosum, genu and splenium, 75
  homolateral to hemiparesis, 72
  patients without paresis, 71
  tetraparesis, 74

G

Glasgow Coma Scale (GCS), 52, 64, 65, 107
  bivariant histogram, 50, 52, 53
  brain stem and thalamus injury rates, 53, 54
  clinical characteristics, 50
  patient distribution, 27, 47–49
  Spearman's rank correlation analysis, 48
Glasgow Outcome Scale (GOS), 26–28, 52, 64
  patient distribution, 47–49
  Spearman's rank correlation analysis, 48

H

Hydrocephalus, 128–129

I

Intracranial pressure (ICP), 13

M

Magnetic resonance imaging (MRI)
  acute TBI, 53, 55–59
  bilateral damages
    medulla oblongata, 53–55, 60–64
    midbrain level, 53, 58
    pons level, 53, 59
  bivariant histogram, 50, 52, 53
  brain stem injury rate, 59, 65
  clinical and prognostic value
    DWI, 7
    1H MR spectroscopy, 7–8
    susceptibility-weighted imaging, 6
    T2-FLAIR, 6
    T2* gradient echo sequences, 6
    T1/T2-weighted imaging, 6
  clinical characteristics, 50
  vs. CT, 61
    acute period of TBI, 35, 36
    corpus callosum damages, 35, 37, 39
    cortical-subcortical focal contusion, 36, 42
    microhemorrhages, 36, 38, 43–46
    patient baseline characteristics, 35, 36

Magnetic resonance imaging (MRI) (*cont.*)
posttraumatic cytotoxic edema,
36, 39–41
subacute subdural hematoma, 36, 42
water diffusion and anisotropy
disturbances, 35, 38–39
mild TBI, 56, 64
MRI data
age groups, corpus callosum injury
rate, 50, 51
brain stem and thalamus injury
rates, 53, 54
causes of TBI, 50, 51
comatose state and unfavorable
outcomes, 53, 54
MRI gradation, 46, 47, 49, 52
patients' age, 46, 47
regional cerebral blood flow
epidural hematoma, 129, 132–133
focal contusion, 129, 132–133, 143,
145–146
primary brain stem damage, 139, 140
subdural hematoma, 130, 133,
138, 139
severe TBI
Firsching's classification, 42, 43
Mannion's analysis, 43
patient distribution, 46–49
sopor, 55, 60–61
Spearman's rank correlation analysis, 48
supratentorial cortical-subcortical
lesions, 53, 55
unilateral damage, midbrain-pons level,
53, 57
Magnetic resonance tomography
apparent diffusion coefficient, 31, 32
corpus callosum, 31, 32
corticospinal tracts, 31–33
diffusion anisotropy, 31
FA value, 31, 32
two-dimensional color-coding maps,
31, 32
Meningoencephalitis, 128–129
Middle cerebral artery (MCA), 108, 119,
120, 130–132
MRI. *See* Magnetic resonance imaging (MRI)

P
Positron emission tomography (PET), 9, 11
Posterior cerebral arteries (PCA), 29, 115,
119, 120, 145
Posterior limb of the internal capsule
(PLIC), 31, 72, 97, 102
Posttraumatic cytotoxic edema, 36, 39–41

R
Regional cerebral blood flow (rCBF)
brain stem, 138
average rCBF values, 143,
144, 152
comatose patients, 139, 142
diffuse axonal injury, 139, 140,
143, 147
diffuse edema and ischemia, 143,
147–148
focal contusions, 143, 145–146, 153
Glasgow Coma Scale, 146, 151, 152
gunshot injury, 139, 141
hemiparesis, 139, 142
increasing ischemia, 145, 147,
149–151
right corticospinal tract, 139
clinical analysis, 125–126
hemispheric brain structures
cerebral perfusion study, 126–128
coma, decompressive craniectomy,
129, 130
corticospinal tract and corpus
callosum, 133, 139
cranioplasty, 129–131
cystic-atrophic changes, 129,
133–135, 138
diffuse axonal injury, 126–129
focal contusion and epidural
hematoma, 129, 132–133
hemorrhagic contusions, 151
meningoencephalitis and
hydrocephalus, 128–129
persistent/increasing ischemia, 129,
134–135
subdural hematoma, 130–131, 133,
135–137

S

Single-photon emission computer tomography (SPECT), 8, 9, 11, 14, 15
Susceptibility-weighted imaging (SWI), 6

W

White matter fiber tracts
   cerebral pathology, 102
   corpus callosum and corticospinal tract condition
     acute period of TBI, 69–74
     dynamic DT-MRI study, 74–101

DAI, 102
interhemispheric interaction, 103
projection pathways, 104
split brain, 103
TBI pathogenesis, 104
tetraparesis, 103

X

Xenon-enhanced CT (XeCT), 11

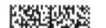